THE COMPLETE GUIDE TO
OUTDOOR WORKOUTS

THE COMPLETE GUIDE TO

OUTDOOR WORKOUTS

Matt Lawrence

BLOOMSBURY

LONDON • NEW DELHI • NEW YORK • SYDNEY

Published by Bloomsbury Publishing Plc
50 Bedford Square
London WC1B 3DP
www.bloomsbury.com

ISBN (print): 978 1 4081 5751 0
ISBN (E-pub): 978 1 4081 8149 2
ISBN (E-pdf): 978 1 4081 8150 8

A CIP catalogue record for this book is available from the British Library.

Acknowledgements
Cover photograph © Corbis Images
Inside photographs © Grant Pritchard
Designed by James Watson
Commissioned by Charlotte Croft
Edited by Sarah Cole

This book is produced using paper that is made from wood grown in managed, sustainable forests. It is natural, renewable and recyclable. The logging and manufacturing processes conform to the environmental regulations of the country of origin.

ViPR, Powerbag, BOSU, Suspension Training®, TRX® and TRX® Rip™ Trainer are all registered trademarks

Typeset in 10.75pt on 14pt Adobe Caslon by seagulls.net

Printed and bound in India by Replika Press Pvt. Ltd.

10 9 8 7 6 5 4 3 2 1

// CONTENTS

PREFACE

When deciding to write this book on outdoor workouts, I wanted to explore a number of factors. Firstly, I wanted to establish who I was writing this book for and who might benefit from reading it. I then revisited many of the training principles, exercises and activities I have utilised with clients in an outdoor environment as a personal trainer, and decided to incorporate a number of more recent training principles and equipment options that I currently use as part of my own training.

With this in mind, and for the integrity of this book, please understand that it would not be possible to incorporate every exercise variation that can be performed with every piece of exercise equipment in the open air. That said, you will hopefully enhance your training programme by applying many of the dynamic and sports-specific drills, functional exercises and workout plans in Parts Two and Three. I have included exercises for all major muscles and, where appropriate, have suggested possible conditioning techniques that encourage balance, agility, speed, strength and power, vital for functional fitness and applicable for many different sports.

Part One gives the reader a brief overview of simple physiology and covers some of the basic fitness principles in preparation for applying these principles in the next two parts of the book.

Part Two identifies specific functional and dynamic warm-up and stretching options, together with sport-related footwork and reactive balance drills to stimulate your motor skills, which will prepare you for many of the workouts to follow.

Part Three, while being of value to fitness enthusiasts and personal trainers alike, also opens itself up to the relatively new exerciser who is not a member of a gym and is simply looking at options for exercising in the outdoors, whether that be at home in the garden, at a park or even at the beach. You might simply begin with fitness walking and potentially move up to jogging as your fitness improves, and you may even get to utilise the Trim Trail options in your local park (see pages 216–223). This section is also applicable to 'new' mothers, with a chapter on buggy workouts, together with a number of other outdoor activities that can be attempted either on your own or with someone else. Part Three is by far the largest section of this book as I wanted to demonstrate working out with minimal equipment in the early chapters before moving forwards to a complete 'tour de force' in chapter 10, which looks at bootcamps, which are suitable for any trainer thinking about setting up or currently running their own programmes. The fitness enthusiast might like the style and diversity of exercise choices offered in bootcamp training and so might be motivated to sign up for a bootcamp class at their local park. For the bootcamp purists out there, I have moved away from the minimalist equipment aspect common to a number of bootcamps, as I have already covered many bodyweight-only exercises in previous chapters. For the purposes of this book, I wanted to highlight the range and complexity of exercises that might be included in a 'professionally run' outdoor workout class.

I have specifically tried to steer away from the more conventional resistance exercises, as I wanted to demonstrate variety in regards to exercise selection and to encourage some lateral thinking in personal trainers and fitness enthusiasts alike. While I have listed certain exercises for use in certain environments, there is no definitive list and obviously there will be a cross over of exercises that can be used in many different environments and locations. After all, there are only a certain number of ways you can lift, pull, push, twist, squat and lunge to create the movement patterns relative to humans. For each workout chapter, I have designed simplistic workout plans, but again these programmes are by no means exhaustive and really only scratch the surface of what might be included, subject to the environment and time available and your fitness level and specific goals.

I hope this book encourages you to explore different options in your training repertoire, whether it is simply to try a new exercise or a complete new workout option, such as using kettlebells or suspension straps. Either way, I hope you will be motivated to try something new as a result of reading this book.

Once you understand the principles of overload and have also got to grips with safe and effective warm-up principles, then the world is your oyster. Only your imagination restricts how you can modify an exercise. The internet has made available thousands of exercise variations and as long as you understand the potential benefits and risks associated with each exercise, then peruse at your will – visit sites such as YouTube, or make use of the many personal trainers creating video downloads that demonstrate their ideas to a mass audience. Be careful though, as sometimes the element of ego overrides the positivity of the exercise choice and it will not be appropriate for all fitness levels, such is the case of the 'look what I can do' syndrome of some 'fitness professionals' showcasing their skills online.

However you decide to utilise this book, please remember that fitness is relative and there are no absolutes with training. In much the same way as you alone can determine what food you find the tastiest, it is also impossible for me to define what training plan is the best for you. Quite simply, the best training plan is the one that works for and is the most enjoyable to you.

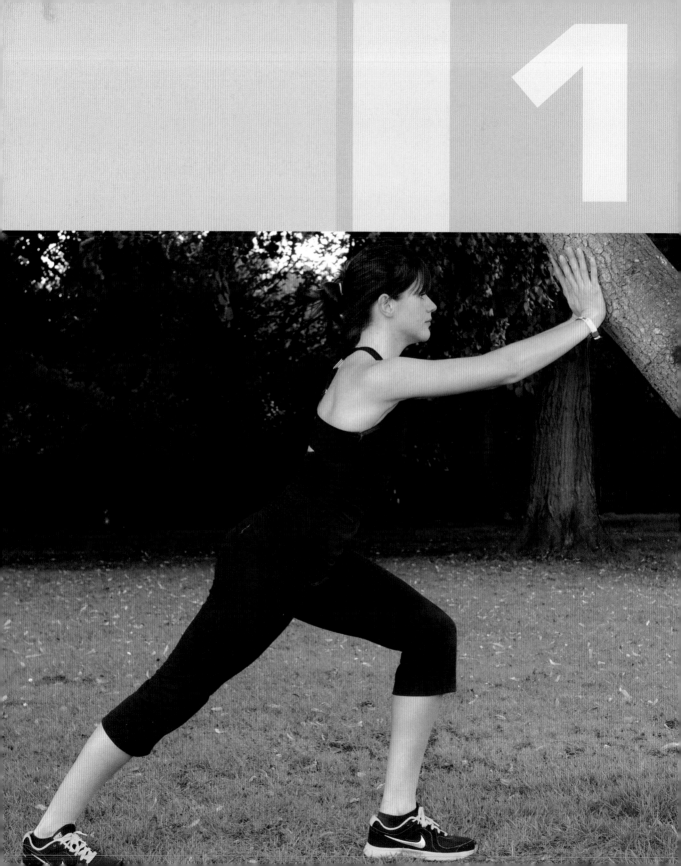

PART **ONE**

EXERCISE PRINCIPLES

BASIC CONDITIONING PRINCIPLES

1

EXERCISE PHYSIOLOGY

Performing any movement or activity requires the heart, lungs and muscles to work at an increased intensity than when at rest, according to the nature and intensity of the activity. With this in mind, your base fitness level will be a factor in the nature of activity you should start with and subsequently progress to, and there are numerous training plans throughout Part Three that can be used as a guide for all fitness levels.

Whatever your reason for exercising, you need to listen to your body and understand your own fitness level. Are you able to walk for a couple of miles but the thought of going for a run gives you the shivers? Might you be able to jog comfortably for 30 minutes but can't perform a single push-up? It is important to understand that whatever your reasons for exercising – weight loss, general fitness, improved health or toning up – by following a suitable training programme you can improve your overall fitness. You can achieve goals if you apply yourself and commit to regular workouts that challenge you, whether you are on your own or working out with others.

When considering a training programme, you should begin with what you can do and work from there, performing the cardio or strength training exercises that you can do safely and effectively under control and gradually increasing the intensity and/or resistance accordingly.

THE CARDIOVASCULAR SYSTEM

Cardiovascular endurance is the body's ability to perform repeated movements over a period of time. The heart is required to pump more blood to the lungs, which oxygenate the blood before it returns to the heart and then it is pumped around the body to supply the muscles, organs and brain. As your heart is a muscle, if it is deconditioned it will have to work harder and beat faster to pump the blood around your body, even for relatively light exercise such as gentle walking. As the intensity of the exercise increases, your heart has to work harder, pumping more blood at a faster rate around your body. In addition, as more oxygen is required, your breathing will become faster and deeper to provide the oxygen that your blood needs to transmit to the muscles. While light to moderate activity can be sustained for relatively long periods through aerobic metabolism (relative to the individual), higher intensity activities cannot be sustained for as long. When the intensity of the activity causes greater oxygen demands from the muscles than can be supplied, you are forced to stop.

Aerobic exercise is exercise that can be maintained with a sufficient amount of oxygen for prolonged periods. This can also be categorised as short (2–8 minutes), medium (8–30 minutes) or long (30 minutes+).[1] Activities that are aerobic in nature are walking, jogging, circuit training, etc. But changes in intensity can push an aerobic activity into becoming *anaerobic* in nature. In this case, to maintain the activity you should reduce the intensity to allow a recovery element. Circuit training is a great aerobic workout with challenging exercises or intervals that push your heart rate up, followed by light active or passive sections which allow you to recover. Higher-intensity activities can be classed as *anaerobic* in nature because the demands of the activity cannot be sustained for long periods. The energy systems used primarily to fuel anaerobic activities differ according to the intensity and duration. For example, sprinting at top speed can only be maintained for a few seconds (8–12) before the intensity has to be reduced, whereas performing activities like shuttle runs or burpees might be maintained for between 30 and 90 seconds, depending on your fitness and the intensity achieved.

INTERVAL TRAINING

The research to promote interval training (repeated intervals of more intense activity interspersed with recovery intervals at a lower intensity) over steady-state training (continuous exercise at the same intensity) is becoming quite overwhelming. However, one has to consider the target audience, together with fitness level and also, to a degree, what the exerciser is actually prepared to do.[2] I am a firm advocate that the most time-effective form of fitness training is undoubtedly interval training, as you can really challenge your aerobic and anaerobic fitness through quite demanding fitness intervals. However, if time is not an issue and your goal is weight loss, for example, this does not have to be the only choice. The simple reality is that whatever you do, in regards to weight loss, it is all about calories consumed versus calories expended over time, not just a specific workout. Within most workout plans, however, it is useful to balance exercises and activities that help train both your aerobic and anaerobic systems for best results.

The intensity-recovery element of interval training really depends on the extent of the intensity – hard/very hard/maximal effort – together with the recovery element – passive/light aerobic/moderate aerobic – and lastly the fitness level of the person in question. In addition, the work/rest ratio might need adjustment when repeated numerous times, i.e. as you perform the third/fourth/fifth/sixth interval etc., your recovery time might need to be longer. Basically, depending upon your fitness and level of intensity reached, the longer the interval, the shorter the recovery as a percentage of the interval.[3]

According to your fitness level, maybe try a rest/work interval of 3:1 for beginners (45 seconds' rest with 15 seconds' work) or for the more advanced 2:1 (30 seconds' rest and 15 seconds' work). For longer work durations of 30 seconds a 2:1 or 3:1 ratio might be appropriate (30 seconds' work: 60–90 seconds' recovery). Or for longer intervals at a slightly lower intensity, a 2:1, 1:1 or even 1:2 ratio might be relative (1 minute's work with 2 minutes, 1 minute or 30 seconds recovery respectively), according to fitness level and exercise intensity (see table 1.1).[4]

Fitness and health benefits

One of the benefits of aerobic exercise is the improved efficiency and capacity of your

Table 1.1	Interval workout example for sports training		
	Distance training	**Mid-distance training**	**Sprint training**
Work/rest ratio	1:1	1:2	1:3
Effort time	5–15 min	30 sec–3 min	10–30 sec
Recovery time	5–15 min	60 sec–6 min	30–90 sec
Repetitions	2–5	5–10	10–20
Aerobic/anaerobic	Aerobic	Anaerobic	Anaerobic

cardiovascular system. The muscles you use to breathe allow you to have a lower, more efficient breathing rate as they become more conditioned. Your heart gets stronger and can pump more blood around your body with each contraction increasing your *stroke volume.*[5] This in turn effects your *cardiac output*, which is your stroke volume multiplied by your heart rate. As more blood is being pumped with each beat, your resting heart rate lowers. Consequently, your heart becomes more efficient both during exercise and while at rest. Aerobic training also benefits the muscles, increasing the size and volume of the *mitochondria* in the muscle cell wall.

Many of the health, fitness and performance benefits of regular aerobic exercise can be seen below:

- Strengthens heart and respiratory muscles
- Reduces blood pressure
- Increases number of red blood cells assisting oxygen transport throughout body
- Reduces risk of diabetes
- Helps to control weight
- Promotes psychological well-being

- Increases bone density (low and high impact weight-bearing activities)
- Improves neuromuscular efficiency
- Increases lean muscle tissue

RESISTANCE TRAINING

Strength training challenges the muscles to respond to a resistance so that they adapt and become stronger. By increasing the resistance and/or variables of overload, this will stimulate the muscles to develop subject to the nature of overload and intensity applied, which is known as '*progressive overload*'.[6] Muscles are stimulated by creating a force on the muscle for it to respond to. This can be through gravity, as when you perform bodyweight exercises or lift dumbbells/kettlebells etc.; using *variable resistance*, such as a resistance tube; or to overcome forces as a result of the movement itself. This might be when using a ViPR (*see* chapter 5, p. 43), throwing a medicine ball, or trying to maintain form while using suspension cables and/or unstable bases.

When you first begin, much of the training will be developing your *motor skills*, essentially learning the movement. However, this sounds easier than it is. If you have never lifted a pair of dumbbells over your head before, sometimes it is not the weight of the dumbbells that causes the problem. You have the strength to lift them but the muscles and stabilising muscles haven't yet learned when and how to contract and with what force. Consequently your movement or motor skill is poor. Through repeated training, you will develop your motor skill and your nerves and muscles will become more efficient, a process called *'neuromuscular adaptation'*.[7]

When you have learned the *movement pattern*, then it is time to progress the overload. You may do this by simply increasing the resistance, but if that is not a simple option (as it might be in a gym with more equipment), you can increase the intensity by adding volume (more sets/repetitions), by reducing the recovery time, or by changing the nature of the exercise (such as the timing of each repetition or even using unstable bases). You can modify the programme itself so that it incorporates more intervals and/or *super-set* exercises, or modify the exercise selection by making the exercises harder, e.g. squats become squat jumps or push-ups become travelling push-ups over a distance etc. This is also true when considering your strength in relation to balanced positions. Combining exercises can also create a whole new perspective for overload. For example, performing a single-arm dumbbell press overhead might be manageable when standing upright but is considerably harder while maintaining the lower position during a forward lunge.

Each muscle has a mix of fast-twitch and slow-twitch fibres and all of us are born with a mix of these fibres. This is part of our genetic make-up and, to a degree, it predetermines who will be able to run the fastest or jump the highest in pure tests where technique or learned skill is not an issue.

Regardless of your genetic make-up, training can help condition your muscles and, subject to your training, intensity, diet and genetics, your muscles will respond accordingly. When performing challenging resistance exercises, there will be a degree of hypertrophy or muscle growth. But to really build bigger muscles, the kind of hypertrophy seen in bodybuilders' physiques, requires very intense conditioning techniques, often using heavy resistances, not just bodyweight. A bodybuilders' workout might include multiple set routines whereby repetitions in the final sets can drop to less than five, focussing on specific muscle groups. Many of the exercises in this book look at functional conditioning techniques, where the repetition range for most exercises is in excess of 15 and thus hypertrophy is not the main focus. The exercises within this book are designed for outdoor workouts and as such the overloads and resistances used will help stimulate the muscles and help create strength and improve general tone, but for greater muscle development and hypertrophy you should really look at training within a gym or health and fitness club, with more equipment and greater resistance to work with.

It is also important to remember the role of flexibility when training with resistance, as all too often the emphasis is on training the muscles for strength and endurance without allowing sufficient recovery and stretching to return the muscle back to its original length. Some of the dynamic stretches demonstrated in Part Two are geared more to the warm-up element of a workout. The appendix (*see* pp. 233–240) also covers self-myofascial release (SMR) techniques to assist in releasing particularly tight muscles, together with more conventional static stretches that might be more appropriate at the end of your workout.

Some of the many benefits of resistance training can be seen below:

- Increased bone density, which helps reduce the onset of osteoarthritis
- Reduced effects of diabetes in some people
- Lowered LDL (low-density lipoprotein) cholesterol
- Improved muscle tone, which can enhance confidence and self-esteem
- Improved posture and reduction in lower back pain
- Improved sleep patterns
- Increased muscle mass, enhancing metabolism and the body's ability to burn fat at rest.

REST DAYS

If you are new to exercise, try and allow a 'rest' day between workouts, which will help you to recover and avoid overtraining and potential injury. If, however, you are an experienced fitness enthusiast, you will probably 'know your body' and how it responds to training – yet even so, always allow one or two lighter or rest days each week.

PROGRAMME DESIGN PRINCIPLES

When designing a programme, a lot depends on your goals, the time you have available and your current fitness level, but rather than just occasionally trying a garden or park workout, a bit more structure is necessary to make the most out of your programme. As a rule, most training programmes incorporate the FITT (Frequency, Intensity, Time, Type) principles, as shown below.

FREQUENCY

This relates to the number of times you exercise over the week or month and is dependent on the time you have available and, to an extent, your goals. If weight loss is your sole objective, the more times over the course of the day/week/month etc. you can exercise, the better, whether your workout is a simple walk or a complete bootcamp-styled workout. However, as with any new activity, you should look to find a healthy balance between training and rest time, so as not to cause injuries through insufficient rest or overuse.

INTENSITY

The intensity or effort level again depends on the objective. For example, when training for a particular sport, the activities and intensities should closely match the sport itself, either directly by developing your skills or indirectly by developing your motor skills, strength and endurance relative to that sport. If weight loss is the goal, then finding a suitable intensity to match that goal is important. There is no point going 'flat out' performing five 25m shuttle runs only to have to sit out the rest of the workout because you are too tired and cannot continue. Always start at a level that you can maintain and increase from there as you begin to learn your fitness limitations. Quite simply, as with all training, don't push too hard, too quickly.

TIME

This is simply how long you train for and is usually a reflection of the time you have available. A two-hour walk on a Sunday morning is great to assist weight loss but walking once a week will not improve your overall fitness. Ideally, you should factor in an additional 20–30 minutes' daily exercise or repeat the two-hour walk 2–3 times per week. Similarly, attending a Saturday morning bootcamp is great, but unless you back it up with activity during the week, you might not achieve your goals as quickly as you want, if at all.

TYPE

The type of exercise is also of importance and while it is important to cross-train to avoid injuries and to give the muscles and joints a recovery, it is equally important to balance muscle groups and intensity sessions when working with resistance or during cardio sessions. From this perspective I would not recommend doing complete full-body workouts on a daily basis, as the muscles need recovery time. If you have the time to train every day, then mix the training up by rotating outdoor workout sessions with walks, runs and even bike rides, and, where possible, always have one rest day or easy day per week.

SUMMARY

- Cardiovascular fitness is the improvement of the heart lungs and muscles through aerobic and/or anaerobic training.
- Aerobic activity involves the large muscle groups and can be maintained for long periods, subject to the intensity.
- Anaerobic training requires working at higher intensities but this cannot be maintained for longer than 1–2 minutes.
- Resistance training can incorporate body-weight, external resistance (dumbbells, ViPRs, etc.) and resistance bands.
- Progressive overload is the graduated increment of various overloads to the exercise or programme over time.
- Progressions should incorporate the FITT principle with regards to overall programme design and development.

FUNCTIONAL CONDITIONING // PRINCIPLES

2

FUNCTIONAL TRAINING

Functional training encourages movement patterns that closely mimic daily life or replicate a specific sporting action. All exercises come from simple movement patterns and include squatting, lunging, pushing, pulling, twisting and bending.[8] How we incorporate these principal movements into varied exercise programmes comes down to the specificity of the sport or activity, together with your fitness, motor-skill ability and neuromuscular integration.

Functional training has its origins in rehabilitation and for a long time the concept was simply a by-product of the therapy room, where it is used to help resolve injuries and movement and/or posture issues. Today, it is widely used in fitness instructing. However, sometimes trainers can get caught up in the 'functional phenomenon', forgetting all else. For example, functional training doesn't mean you have to hang from a suspension cable performing modified pull-ups with your feet on a BOSU (unless you need to perform similar movements within your sport, such as for kite-surfing or windsurfing perhaps).

Functional movement should be multi-planar in nature (movement in three planes of motion) as opposed to a single plane of motion, which is often the case when using conventional gym equipment. The different planes and their relevant actions can be seen in table 2.1.

For an exercise to be fully functional it should reflect a lifestyle activity or a specific sporting movement. To explain this further, when training your legs, while the seated leg-press machine might be great for developing pure leg strength in this position, the extent to how much of this strength is transferable to life situations is questionable. A better choice would be a split-stance dumbbell squat which replicates the functionality of sitting down or reaching down to pick something up. This can be progressed functionally by lunging forward to pick up two dumbbells, in a modified split-stance position, then standing up holding the dumbbells and finally stepping forwards to place them down on the floor again. This pick up/put down technique has a purpose relative to life movements and so has a functional perspective.

FUNCTIONAL CONDITIONING PROGRESSION

From a training perspective, functional movements should begin with bodyweight exercises moving through various planes of motion. Then introducing a stabilisation requirement, additional

Table 2.1   Planes of motion

Plane of motion	Motion/action	Example
Sagittal plane	Flexion/extension	Walking, squatting, biceps curl, frontal raise
Frontal plane	Adduction/abduction Side flexion	Jumping jack, air jack, lateral raise, side bending
Transverse plane	Rotation (interior and exterior) Horizontal flexion/extension	Abdominal woodchop, golf swing, reverse flye

resistance and finally dynamic power.[9] This is more applicable to sports, as most sports require movements in all directions.

Using the principles above, take a functional movement like a squat, because every day you will replicate this movement by sitting on a chair, for example. When you can perform a squat with correct technique, challenge your stabilisation within the movement, such as by squatting while on a BOSU (*see* chapter 5, p. 42). This helps train your proprioceptive system, which analyses how balanced you are and which muscles to contract to keep your balance, and will improve *total body integration*, i.e. the involvement of all nerves, muscles, joints and ligaments working together to perform a specific movement. When you can squat with good form on a BOSU, introduce resistance without using the BOSU and squat using a barbell or holding dumbbells. As your movement becomes competent then reintroduce the BOSU and perform the squat using the extra resistance before gradually applying dynamic speed under control.

To improve your jump, you would need to train your motor skills, nerves and muscles, collectively to improve your jump height. You should incorporate functional jump-related exercises, which could include resisted jumps using weighted vests and resisted jumping from unstable bases in which the movement patterns resemble the end movement. In this way you train the nerves and muscles in a directly similar way to the desired movement.

THE KINETIC CHAIN

Mobility and flexibility are the building blocks of strength, speed, power endurance and agility.[10] Physical performance is about movement development and, while previous training principles have focused on training muscles in isolation, often for hypertrophy, the current focus is to train the movement rather than the muscle. Rather than focus on *isolation exercises*, functional training trains muscles and joints '*holistically*', integrating groups of muscles and joints throughout a movement that challenges your balance, improves your stabilisation and develops your co-ordination. Consider walking up stairs carrying a heavy load – the increased weight might throw your natural centre of gravity out slightly, causing you to have to adjust your stance or movement to stay balanced. If this fails at any point, you might need to hold on to the wall or take a step back. This 'neuromuscular awareness' can be trained to improve, and as the muscles of the trunk are required for all upright postures, training on an unstable base can assist your *stabiliser* and *neutraliser* muscles to respond rapidly, improving your balance and co-ordination. The science behind this holistic or integrated training process starts with understanding the *kinetic chain*.

The kinetic chain is an integrated functional unit comprising muscles, tendons, ligaments, fascia, nerves and bones.[11] All these elements need to work in harmony for optimum movement and performance. This synergy of working together is known as *neuromuscular efficiency*. Where there are imbalances within this unit, problems can occur, such as decreased performance, muscle trauma or even injury. If one muscle group is weak, other muscles might have to compensate to maintain a movement; this is known as 'synergistic dominance'.[12] An example of this might be where certain gym enthusiasts over-train their chest muscles, with little time spent training their back; the result being short tight chest muscles and long weak back muscles. This imbalance disrupts the efficiency of the neuromuscular system and the kinetic chain is compromised. It is necessary to try and recondition the weakened muscle through appropriate training to help restore the balance in the kinetic chain.

FUNCTIONAL TRAINING EQUIPMENT

Functional fitness programmes often involve the use of balance or unstable training methods while performing an exercise or activity using an additional overload. Equipment used in functional fitness exercises might include some or all of the following (*see also* chapter 5, pp. 41–44):

- Cable machine
- Stability ball
- Wobble board/Reebok core board/rocker board/ BOSU/balance disc
- Resistance tubes
- Kettlebells
- Suspension Training® systems
- TRX® Rip™ Trainer
- Sandbag/Powerbag
- ViPR
- Medicine ball
- Dumbbells
- Club/hammer/rope/tyre

FUNCTIONAL CONDITIONING FOR SPORTS

Functional strength is the ability to apply your strength in an environment that is more relative to the action or movement in your required sport.[13] For the sports enthusiast, *functional strength* is important, but there is a big difference between *absolute strength* – your ability to lift a specific weight from a stable environment such as a bench press – and transferable or functional strength. Functional strength is determined according to the amount of force or power you can apply relative to the demands of the activity or sport.

- **Power** is about exerting force against a resistance or object. This requires a strong core and integration of muscles and joints to apply the force within a movement. This would occur when you dynamically step upwards on to a step or bench, leap off a rock or jump over a breakwater during a beach workout.
- **Speed** is fundamental in sports, but while pure speed is only relative in events such as the 100m or 200m events in athletics, acceleration and the ability to pass an opponent or

competitor is useful in nearly all other sports, such as football or rugby. This focuses on your ability to change pace and add intensity, together with your agility, weight shift and rapid direction change.

- **Agility** is about applying acceleration and deceleration relative to your sport. Having the ability to change direction at speed involves a number of biomechanical considerations, together with adjustments in speed, power, strength, co-ordination, dynamic balance and dynamic stabilisation. In sport you need to be able to change direction, stop, rotate, jump and leap, often repeatedly, without losing your body position or form.

- **Co-ordination** can cover many aspects, and while this skill is imperative to enhance your overall development, the nature of the sport or activity will dictate the extent of your motor-skill development.

- **Reactions** are extremely important in all sports, whether responding to adjustments in the terrain you are running on or encountering an environment that you have not planned for, such as a stray dog deciding it wants to join in your shuttle run in a park workout.

- **Balance** is often associated with agility, yet it does not actually have to involve movement. From a functional perspective, balance is very important when holding a position while performing a specific exercise or movement, such as stand-up paddleboarding or martial arts. Yet balance becomes far more important in specific sporting applications.

- **Proprioception** is the way that the body reacts and recovers from being unbalanced. Any external force, such as gravity, a strong wind or an unstable floor, can cause the body to lose its balance ability for a moment. The muscles are constantly providing feedback to the brain about their surroundings and forces acting on them. The brain sends messages via the nerves to the muscles on how to respond and when. This two-way process of internal feedback using sensory awareness and muscle and joint sensitivity creates this complex system of 'proprioception'.[14]

Functional training should always be geared towards an end goal. For example, within a sports context you should integrate appropriate equipment and stabilisation techniques that help to mimic the specific sporting movement. Then challenge these movements by increasing the stabilisation required to help integrate the muscles and develop functional strength, relative to the sporting movement. If sport is not the main focus then any exercise that incorporates multi-planar movement with varying levels of graduated stability and resistance can be applied as appropriate.

SUMMARY

- Exercises should be based on life movements or sporting actions relative to the individual, the nature of the sport and their ability.
- Training programmes should be individualised so that they are geared to training the specific needs of the individual.
- Programmes should be integrated and progressive using a variety of multi-planar exercises and with appropriate overload to develop movement with increased flexibility, enhanced core strength, muscular strength and power, together with improved balance.

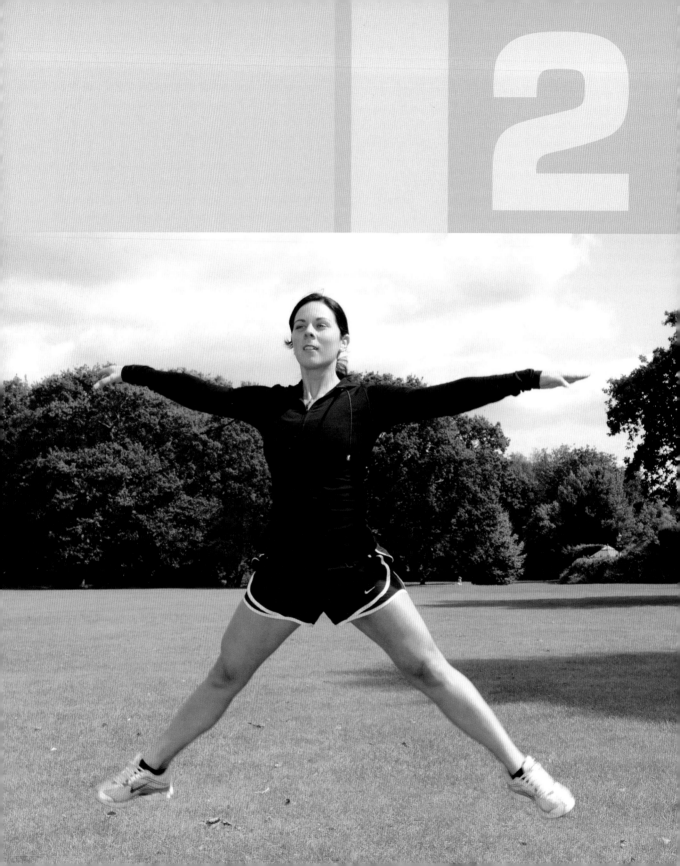

PART **TWO**

WARMING UP PRINCIPLES AND GUIDELINES

FUNCTIONAL WARM-UPS

3

WARMING UP

While in the past static stretching formed the basis of most warm-ups, recent research has suggested that it is important that the muscle is warm and has been taken through its full range of movement relative to the activity to follow.[15] The incidence of injury has been shown to be greatly reduced when the warm-up is performed appropriately and relatively according to the sport.[16] Activities and movements within your warm-up should replicate the nature of the following activity, albeit at a lower intensity. If your workout is to go for a run, then warm up by walking and light jogging. If you are intending to work out with weights, you should mobilise the joints and perform exercises or movements that take the joints through similar movement patterns to your workout routine.[17] This should begin with light resistance to stimulate the muscles.

A warm-up should also prepare your body for aerobic and even anaerobic activity, by placing demands on your cardiovascular system to increase your heart rate and consequently assist oxygen transportation via the bloodstream to the muscles.

Movements should also be rhythmic and dynamic in nature and allow for sufficient progression in intensity, helping to reduce the risk of injury. For example, if you are beginning a sprint training session, you should include sprints as part of your warm-up, but at a reduced yet progressive intensity. After performing many of the warm-up techniques demonstrated later in this section, you should incorporate some acceleration movements to include progressive sprint drills, starting at a comfortable speed – perhaps 30–50 per cent intensity – and building up gradually to 80–85 per cent intensity.

Warming up for a multi-movement sport, such as football, tennis or rugby, should involve a far more varied repertoire of movement, twists, turns, accelerations, sprints and jumps as part of the preparation for the game itself. While this book does not focus on these sports, many of the dynamic warm-up drills, together with the footwork and agility drills in chapter 4, will assist your motor-skill development relative to many sports.

It is also important following a workout or activity session that adequate time is spent cooling down. A cool-down effectively allows the body to dissipate waste products such as lactic acid and reduces the chances of blood pooling, light headedness and/or muscle cramps. Blood pooling is simply when the blood is not being pumped around the body sufficiently and during intense exercise, stopping abruptly would not allow de-oxygenated blood to be pumped back to the heart adequately. In addition, cooling down reduces the amount of adrenaline in the blood and allows a safe time to return your heart rate to normal.

The following selection of functional warm-up exercises incorporates dynamic movements and stretches, and it is important to graduate your

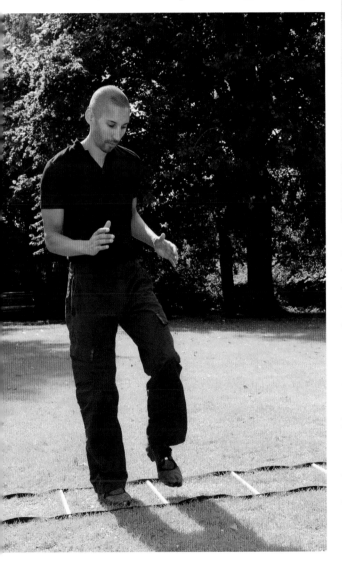

Static versus dynamic stretching

The case for static pre-stretching as opposed to dynamic stretching is still open, yet arguably dynamic movement that takes the muscle through its full range safely and relative to the movements required within the sport is far more appropriate. My only concern, having worked with numerous enthusiasts of all fitness levels and varying body awareness, is that sometimes it is useful to incorporate a static stretching element in your warm-up, as often some enthusiasts do not have the movement quality to achieve a suitable stretch through dynamic movement alone. In these situations, providing it is not detrimental to the warm-up process, I would suggest that static stretches of the hamstrings and calf muscles have their place.

speed and/or nature of movement as you progress through the list. You can perform as many as you wish, depending on the nature and intensity of the workout to follow. For sports enthusiasts, I would recommend performing the majority in the order shown, but for the general enthusiast the importance is that you warm up safely by mobilising your joints, increasing your heart rate and incorporating full-body movements to prepare you for your workout. From that perspective, feel free to pick and choose from the exercises provided, making sure that by the end, you feel warm and energised, and that your muscles and joints are ready to work!

Ex 3.1 Arm rotations/circles

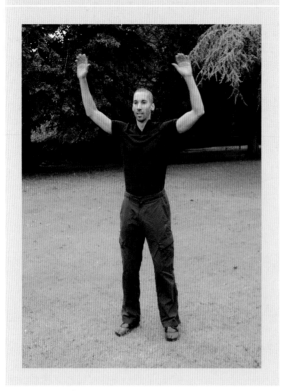

Modifications

- Keep your arms bent with hands near your shoulders to reduce the movement arc, yet still rotate your elbows in a circular movement past your ears and head.
- Alternatively, you can perform the movement with alternate arms in a 'backstroke' technique, one arm after the other.
- You can also rotate both your arms in a forward direction, repeating as before.
- To challenge your co-ordination, you can rotate one arm backwards while rotating the opposite arm forwards. In this case aim for 10–15 rotations before reversing the movement direction for each arm and repeating.

Starting position and action

- Stand upright in a neutral stance and with your arms by your sides.
- Slowly lift both arms forwards, past your ears and over your head in a circle, and back down to your sides.
- Initially, circle your arms around slowly a few times before gradually increasing speed to a more dynamic action.
- Repeat circles 10–15 times.

Ex 3.2 Trunk rotations

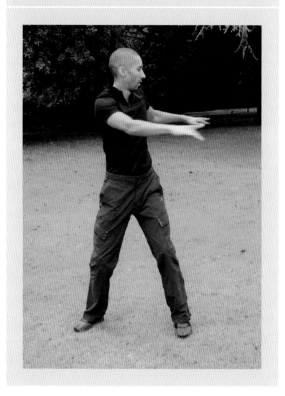

Modifications
- A useful variation of this rotation movement is to add a weight shift from right leg to left leg as you rotate, so that when rotating to the right and reaching across with your left arm, you step further to your right, shifting all your bodyweight to your right leg as you come up on to your toes for balance on your left leg.
- Then repeat the movement to your left, stepping out and shifting your bodyweight to your left, as your right arm reaches across, coming up on to the toes of your right foot.

Starting position and action
- Begin standing upright, with your feet wider than shoulder-width apart, and slowly rotate to your right and then to your left, gradually increasing your range with each twist.
- As you increase your movement range, reach across your chest with your left arm when rotating to your right, allowing your hips to twist and your knees to move slightly. The twisting action will force you to come up on to the toes of your left foot.
- Repeat alternate movements 15–20 times.

Ex 3.3 Up-and-over squats

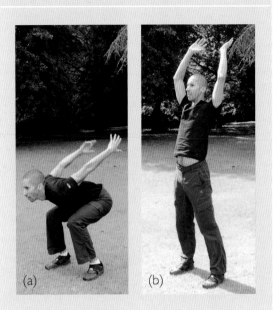

(a) (b)

Ex 3.4 Walking

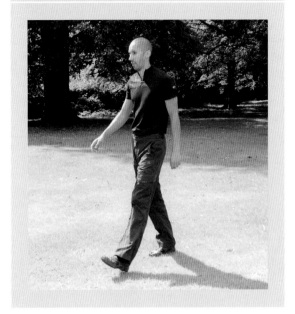

Starting position and action

- Begin with your feet shoulder-width apart and knees slightly bent.
- Flex your knees and hips in a squatting action to bend forwards, bringing your chest towards your thighs and both arms behind you (3.3a).
- Then stand back up, extending your knees and hips, and reach over your head with your arms slightly behind you in a partially hyperextended position (3.3b).
- Repeat this squatting and standing movement between 10 and 15 times.

Starting position and action

- Stand erect with shoulders relaxed and your spine in neutral alignment.
- Begin walking forwards with an exaggerated heel-toe action to loosen the ankle joint and dynamically stretch the muscles of the lower leg.
- Continue walking for about 30 seconds to 1 minute before reversing the action and walking backwards.
- Keep your arms comfortably relaxed and slightly bent throughout.

Ex 3.5 Heel/tip-toe walking

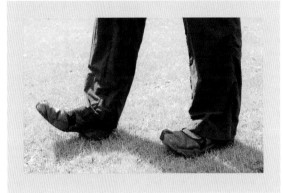

Starting position and action

- Begin standing with feet hip-distance apart and dorsiflex your feet, lifting your toes upwards to take your weight on to your heels.
- Take a step forwards to land on the heel of your right leg but do not allow your foot to roll through as in a normal walking action.
- Instead, immediately step forward with your left foot to land again on the heel of your left leg.
- Continue this heel walking action for 15–20m.
- Then step forwards with your right leg to land on your toes and forefoot and immediately step forward with your left leg, continuing to walk forwards on the balls of your feet and your toes for 15–20m
- Combine this heel-toe walking combination for about a minute.

Ex 3.6 Walking high-knee hugs

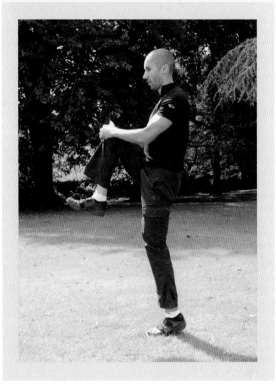

Starting position and action

- Stand upright and begin walking slowly forwards, starting with your left foot first.
- Take three steps and then lift your right knee up and pause briefly as you pull this knee towards your chest, holding your shin with both hands as you do so.
- Release your leg and take three steps before lifting your left knee up, taking hold of your leg with your hands to pull the knee slightly up towards your chest.
- Release and repeat this knee-hugging action every third pace over a distance of 20–30m.
- Repeat this distance 2–3 times.

Ex 3.7 Hip-rotation walk

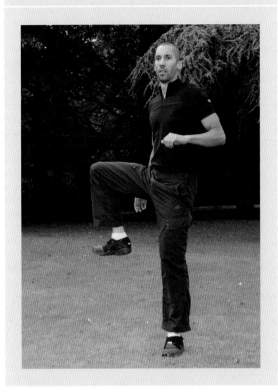

Starting position and action

- This exercise helps to mobilise the hip joint.
- Walk forward for three paces and on the third pace, lift your leg, driving upwards with your knee, and when your thigh is almost parallel with the floor, outwardly rotate your knee before placing your leg back on the floor and continuing to walk forward another three paces.
- On the third pace lift your other knee and rotate outwards before placing your foot back on the floor.
- Repeat these 1, 2, 3, rotations for 10–20m.

Ex 3.8 Hamstring hurdle sprint drills

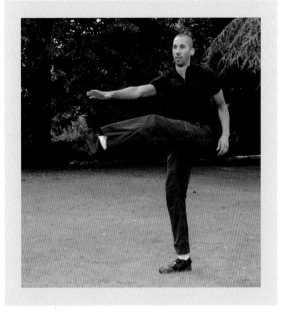

Starting position and action

- Begin walking forward as in exercise 3.7 and on the third pace step forward with a high knee lift, lifting your left knee to hip height with a bent leg. Then, in this position, extend your left leg, maintaining your knee lift to stretch the hamstrings of your left leg.
- From this extended position, lower the left leg to the floor to continue to walk forward, stepping with your left leg, then right, then left and lift your right knee upwards to hip height, extending your right leg to dynamically stretch the hamstrings.
- Follow this extension, bringing your leg to the floor to continue walking.
- Repeat this walk, walk, walk, dynamic stretch technique for 20–30m.

Ex 3.9 Jogging

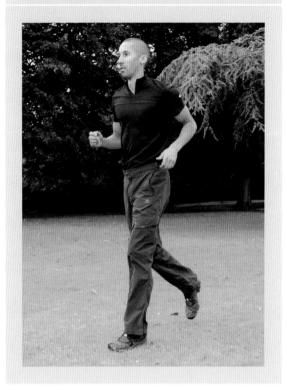

Modifications

- After about 30 seconds to 1 minute of gentle jogging, start to jog backwards, taking shorter paces.
- When jogging backwards, you will land on your forefoot and push off.
- Backward running brings the hamstrings into play, so keep your pace slow initially, remaining upright and not trying to lean either forwards or backwards.
- After about 15–30 seconds of backward running, jog forwards again and repeat for another 10–20 seconds before introducing backward running again.
- In most team and field/court sports the movements are multi-directional, so it is often useful to introduce a combination of forward and backward running and lateral shuffles, together with direction changes and even reaction changes.

Starting position and action

- Begin jogging forwards slowly and gently, absorbing the impact of your landing forces by 'rolling' through the landing in a heel-toe action.
- Take small strides initially before increasing to a normal, slow jogging pace and stride length.
- Keep your arms loose but in a natural jogging action throughout.

Ex 3.10 Skipping

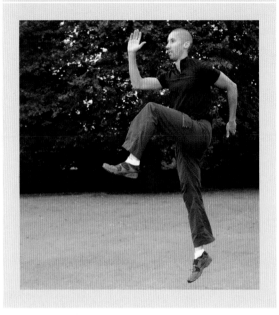

Starting position and action

- This is a compromised running action in that you have a change in rhythm as your feet strike the ground, so that you have a very short stride followed by a long stride where you push yourself into the air.
- Essentially, try to have 'air time' by 'launching' yourself into the air every second stride, contacting the ground twice with your right leg, followed by twice with your left leg etc.
- As your feet hit the ground, push off your second leg to 'hang' in the air before contacting the ground again.
- Continue this skipping technique, aiming to increase your height in the lift and driving your lifted bent knee into the air each time.
- Dynamically swing your arms to assist your 'air time'.

Ex 3.11 Carioca

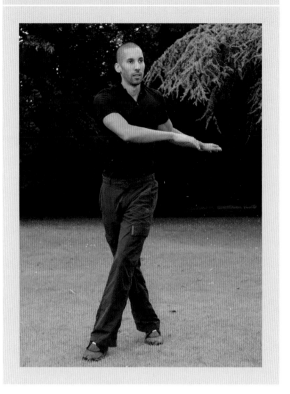

Starting position and action

- This is a co-ordinated lateral stepping action whereby one foot crosses in front and then behind the other as you move to the side.
- Begin with feet hip-distance apart, knees slightly bent and arms by your sides.
- Take your left foot across and in front of your right foot, to take your weight on the ball of your left foot.
- Then step out to the side with your right foot, about 30cm.
- Then lift your left foot and take it behind your right foot, causing you to rotate at your waist slightly.

- Then step out to the right again, before stepping across and in front of your right foot with your left.
- Repeat this front and back cross-over heading to your right for 20–30m before resting briefly and repeating the sequence to your left, this time with your right foot crossing in front and behind your left.
- To assist upright balance and stability, move counter to the twisting action·in order to keep your upper torso facing forwards.
- Repeat 2–3 times.

Ex 3.12 Lateral side-steps/shuffles

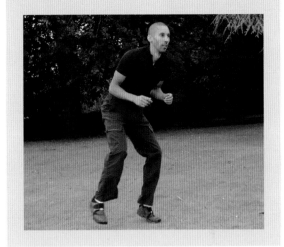

Starting position and action

- Standing upright, keep your knees slightly bent and abdominals braced throughout.
- Step out to the side with your right foot approximately 30–50cm to your right, touching the ground with the balls of your feet.
- As your right foot touches the ground, lift your left foot and bring it a similar distance to the right.
- Then lift your right foot again, placing it 30–50cm to the right, repeating by lifting your left foot to bring yourself back to a neutral stance.
- Continue this lateral shuffle on the balls of your feet with knees slightly bent over a distance of 10–20m before reversing the direction (still facing the same way) to travel back, this time leading the shuffle with your left leg and travelling to your left, to complete the distance back to your start point.
- Rest briefly, before repeating 3–5 times.

Ex 3.13 Graduated dynamic leg swings

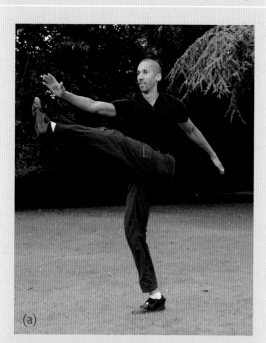

(a)

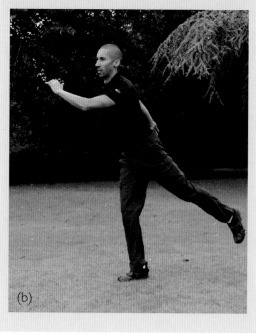

(b)

Starting position and action

- Stand with your feet hip-distance apart and take your weight on to your left leg.
- Begin slowly and under control by gently swinging your right leg forwards and backwards, increasing in height until your right leg nears horizontal position at the top part of the swing.
- On the backward swing do not try to lift the leg too far – rather just far enough to allow the swinging momentum to occur.
- As you lift your right leg towards the horizontal position, try and slow the 'swinging action' down to momentarily pause the movement, maintaining a straight leg throughout.
- Repeat, gradually increasing the range of movement but not so as to compromise your straight leg or body position.
- As you lift your right leg up towards the horizontal position (or higher), reach forwards with your left hand to touch your right foot.
- Repeat for 15–20 swings before changing legs.

Ex 3.14 Forward lunges with double-arm sweep

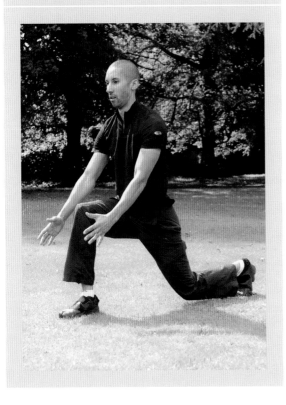

- Repeat the lunge with your other leg, reaching or sweeping forwards with both hands past your front foot as you reach the full lunge position.
- Push back off your front foot to return to a standing position with your arms by your sides.
- Repeat this 'sweeping' alternate lunge movement 15–20 times.

Modifications

- Use a single arm reach so that when you lunge forward with your right leg, you reach down with your left hand towards your right foot.
- Repeat alternate lunges with opposing arm reaches/touches for 20–30 repetitions.

Starting position and action

- Stand erect with feet hip-distance apart and your spine in neutral alignment.
- Step into a forward lunge, keeping both arms by your sides.
- As you bend your front leg going into the lunge, reach or 'sweep' forwards with both hands, bending forwards at your hips so that your hands 'sweep' past your front foot.
- Push back off your front foot, contracting your glutes and thighs to return to a standing position with feet hip-distance apart.

Ex 3.15 Speed skater

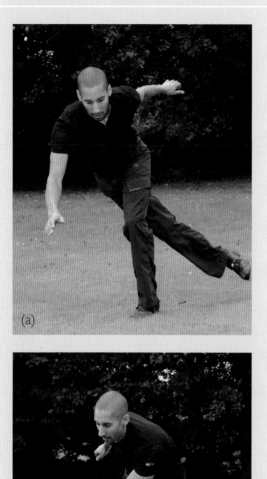

(a)

(b)

Starting position and action

- Begin standing with your feet shoulder-width apart, your knees bent and leaning forward slightly at your hips.
- Keeping your abdominals braced with your hands in front of your chest, dynamically step out approximately 1.5m to your right in a leaping action to balance on your right leg.
- As you do this your left leg follows in a leaping action, but sweeps behind your right leg, initially to tap behind with your toes to assist balance.
- Then dynamically leap/step back to your left to land on your left leg as your right leg follows and you touch the floor behind your left leg with your toes of you right foot.
- Repeat these lateral hops, but increase in both distance and knee flexion as you land to lean forward into a modified 'speed skater' action with your arms swinging naturally to assist both movement and balance.
- As you progress, do not touch behind with your trail leg but keep it in the air so that you are only ever balancing on one leg at a time, with alternate right and left lateral leaps/hops.

Ex 3.16 Iron cross

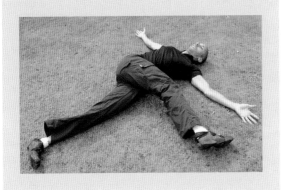

Ex 3.17 Scorpion leg twists

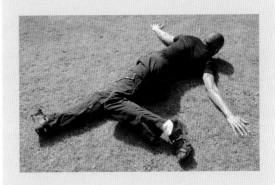

Starting position and action

- Lie on your back with arms out to the side in a crucifix position and your legs together.
- Lift your right leg, keeping abdominals braced, and rotate at your hips to take the leg towards your left hand on the floor.
- Touch the floor with your right foot, just below your left hand, and then return your right leg back to the starting position.
- Now do the same again, this time taking your left leg up towards your right outstretched hand.
- Repeat 5–8 times each side.

Starting position and action

- Lie face down in a crucifix position with arms at right angles to your torso, palms down.
- Then lift your right leg, leading from your heel, and by bending your leg and twisting at the waist, try and bring your right heel over in the direction of your left hand.
- Return the right leg to the start position on the floor and repeat movement, this time taking your left foot towards your right hand, twisting at the waist and with leg bent.
- Avoid trying to overstretch in the movement and repeat 3–5 times on each side.

REACTIVE BALANCE AND LADDER DRILLS

4

REACTIVE BALANCE DRILLS

As part of the warm-up process, it is important to stimulate your reactive balance and co-ordination as this helps to focus the mind and muscles in harmony. This can then benefit your overall workout or, if part of a sports warm up, assist your movement control and performance within the sport itself.

Dynamic balance is the ability to keep your body under control during movement.[18] This might be by maintaining balance while on an unstable base or within a specific agility movement drill.

Reactive balance exercises aim to challenge your neuromuscular responses to a change in body shift and landing forces.[19] Essentially, it is the ability to maintain your balance when you have to adjust after stepping on an object you were not anticipating. The awkward foot placement sends nerve impulses to the brain, which returns impulses to the muscles, encouraging them to react so that you regain balance and control of movement. This 'self-righting' effect can be learned through reactive balance training.

Conventional balance requires you to maintain your centre of gravity over a base of support. Reactive balance exercises aim to challenge your response to landing when your centre of gravity moves from one base of support to another, for example multiple hops to balance. You might want to challenge your balance by jumping on to an unstable base, such as a BOSU or jumping from an unstable base to the floor. Another option is walking on uneven terrain, such as rocks, sand or pebbles. This challenges your proprioception skills and your dynamic and neuromuscular balance. As with the ladder drills (*see* p. 34), it is important to challenge your motor skills and reactive balance early on in the workout, and so include one or two different drills towards the end of your warm-up. Alternatively, incorporate some reactive drills in your workout, within the main circuit or following a high-intensity exercise, providing an active recovery.

Ex 4.1 Forward jumps

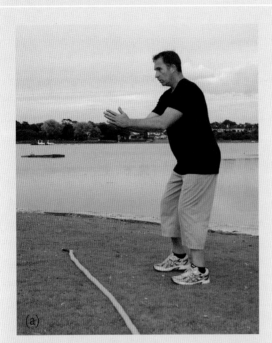

(a)

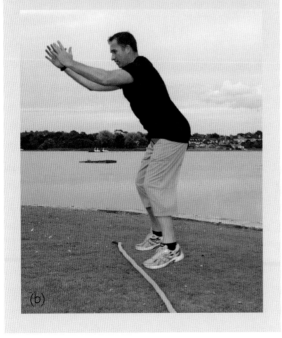

(b)

Starting position and action

- Stand with your feet shoulder-width apart in a neutral stance, with your knees slightly bent and your hips slightly flexed in a 'ready' position.
- With your arms slightly bent and by your sides, swing your arms back as you bend your legs further into a partial squat position.
- Before reaching a full squat, rapidly swing both your arms forwards, with arms bent, pushing off through your legs to jump upwards and forwards.
- Immediately bend your knees and flex at your hips to cushion your landing by squatting down to decelerate and absorbing the impact.
- Aim to land in the same neutral stance as your take-off, with feet shoulder-width apart.
- Pause briefly when you have fully decelerated the landing and then extend your legs to stand back up.
- On completion, walk back to the start position and repeat.
- Repeat forward jumps 5–10 times.
- The emphasis on this exercise is not the height or distance but rather the control on your landing.

Ex 4.2 Horizontal jumps

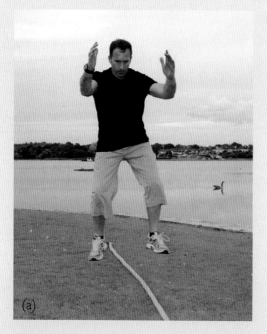

(a)

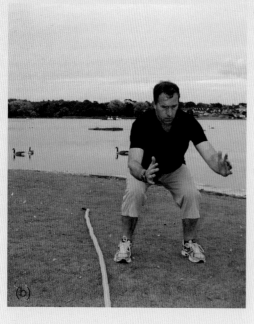

(b)

Starting position and action

- Stand with your feet shoulder-width apart in a neutral stance, but this time when you jump, push off to your right side to land between 30cm and 1m to your right, cushioning your landing by bending your knees.
- Repeat the horizontal jump, this time to your left. Perform 3–5 jumps each side.

Modification: Multi-planar jump

- Begin as before, but when you push off your legs, twist slightly with your torso to your right, in the direction to which you will be jumping.
- Jump out to your right side, rotating to land with your feet shoulder-width apart, between 45 and 135 degrees from your starting position.
- Perform another jump, this time rotating back to your left, either fully to return to the start position or to another point, having rotated/ jumped further or less than your original jump.
- Repeat multi-planar jumps for 8–12 repetitions in total, placing the emphasis on control of jump, focussing on ankle, knee, hips and shoulder stabilisation throughout.

Ex 4.3 Jumps up

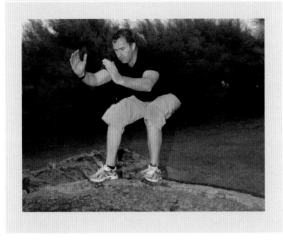

Starting position and action
- Begin facing a bench, log or tree stump, feet hip-distance apart, legs and arms slightly bent.
- Keeping your arms bent, pull them backwards as you lower down into a partial squat before rapidly driving your arms forwards and upwards while extending your legs to jump up on to the bench or log.
- As you jump, lift your knees upwards, flexing through your hips so your feet land shoulder-width apart.
- As you land in the squat position, pause briefly before standing up straight.
- Step down carefully and return to your start position. Repeat for 6–10 jumps.

Modifications
- Add a rotation to the movement while in the air, to land at 45–180 degrees to your original position.
- A word of caution: do not attempt to jump too high as you run the risk of injury if you don't land properly.

Ex 4.4 Drop jumps

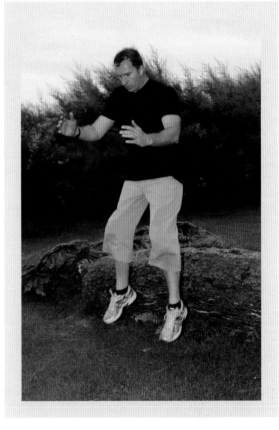

Starting position and action
- This drill is similar to exercise 4.3, except you are jumping down from a height, such as a park bench, wall or even a fallen tree.
- The key is to absorb your landing by decelerating. Bend your knees and hips and squat down to a half-squat position, with feet shoulder-width apart as you land.
- Step back up on to the bench or log and position yourself as before, ready to jump off, repeating 5–10 times.
- Variations would include adding a quarter or half turn to the movement while in the air.

Ex 4.5 Forward steps to balance

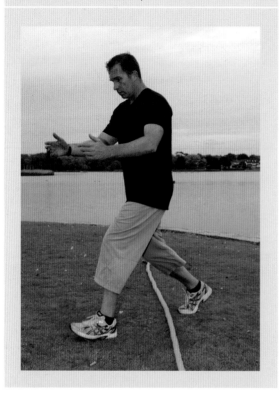

Starting position and action

- Stand upright with your feet hip-distance apart, and your arms by your side.
- Take a large step forwards with your right leg and as you land, lift your left leg to follow but keep it in the air, with your left thigh almost parallel to the floor and your left knee bent at 90 degrees.
- Hold this single balance for 3–5 seconds before lowering your left leg and stepping back, before repeating.
- Try 5–10 steps with your right leg before repeating the exercise, stepping forwards with your left leg.

Modifications

- This exercise can be made more dynamic so that instead of stepping, you leap forwards from a neutral stance, feet hip-distance apart, to land on your right foot, bringing your left leg forward and bent at right angles as before, as you balance on your right leg.
- Take this dynamic step or leap forwards with your right leg, to hold a balance position, but then dynamically step/leap backwards with your left leg to land on your left leg, lifting your right leg with knee bent to 90 degrees.
- Repeat this forward/backward leap for 5–10 repetitions before changing your lead leg, this time leaping forwards on to your left leg.
- In addition to forward and backward steps or leaps, this exercise can be intensified further by adding rotation to the movement to step/leap into the transverse plane.
- In this movement, you would leap forwards on to your right leg, but then rotate your left leg at the hip to point behind you to your left.
- Perform these multi-planar leaps with alternate legs for 10–20 repetitions.

Ex 4.6 Forward hops to balance

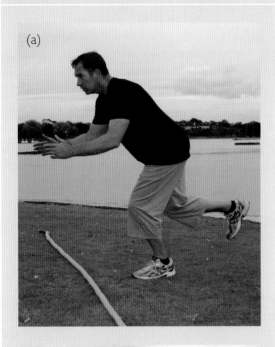

(a)

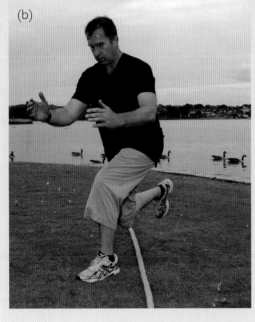

(b)

Starting position and action

- Stand on your right leg with both knees bent slightly and with your arms by your sides.
- Lean forward slightly to maintain your balance and bend further with your right leg before swinging your arms upwards to assist your hopping action.
- As you do so, push off your right leg and hop approximately 1m forwards to land on your right leg, bending your knee to cushion your landing as you do so.
- Ensure as you land that your ankle, knee, hips and shoulders are stabilised, with your abdominals braced and spine in neutral alignment to maintain your balance.

Modification 1:
Horizontal hops to balance

- Begin standing on your right leg as before.
- Push off your right leg to hop approximately 0.5–1m to your right and absorb your impact by bending your leg while maintaining your balance.

Modification 2:
Multi-planar hops to balance

- Begin as before, but this time hop approximately 1m in varied directions, ensuring that as you land you maintain your balance on a single leg for 5 seconds before hopping in a different direction.
- Repeat multi-planar hops for 5–10 repetitions before changing legs and repeating.

Further Modifications

While exercises will train your reactive balance and emphasise joint stability and proprioception, to progress these you could try introducing unstable bases, either to start from, land on to or even both. The forward or horizontal jumps could be on to or off a BOSU, or for a very advanced variation, from one BOSU on to another. As with all exercise progressions, begin with what you can do safely, with effective technique before progressing further.

LADDER DRILLS

Ladder drills are often used as the next stage following a warm-up, before beginning your main workout. They are an excellent way of awakening your motor skills and increasing your heart rate, ready for a sports or dynamic workout. But ladder drills can also be utilised within a main workout to challenge your co-ordination and agility, which are important in many sports, and together with an appropriate strength and conditioning programme, are fundamental preparation when training for a specific sport. For many sports, pure speed is not the key factor (other than a 100m race), but rather acceleration and agility. To achieve the best acceleration you need to have a low centre of gravity and you need to drive forwards with your arms and legs, pumping your knees with a high knee lift and powerful push-off. Having the ability to increase your stride rate, knee lift and push-off is extremely useful.

You can perform numerous speed drills using various sports-specific equipment, such as speed ladders, cones, hurdles and bungee cords, and many of these have been fused into some of the other workouts in Part 3. The emphasis when performing these drills should be on quality of movement and execution. It is better to perform the ladder drills five times with perfect execution than ten times with poor movement quality. The following principles should be maintained when participating in speed drills:

- Avoid unnecessary forward lean at the waist.
- Stay on the balls of your feet.
- Keep your arms pumping fast, with your elbows close to your ribs.
- Stay balanced and remain in a relaxed upright position.

Here are some simple examples of speed and agility drills using ladders that will be of benefit to your warm-up process or can even be used as an interval/agility option within an outdoor workout session. You can choose to perform one or two of the drills, or even complete all of them but, most importantly, ensure you complete them at an intensity that will not cause you to fatigue before the main workout.

Ex 4.7 One foot in

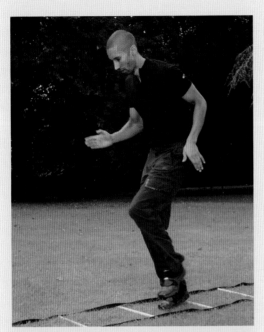

Modification

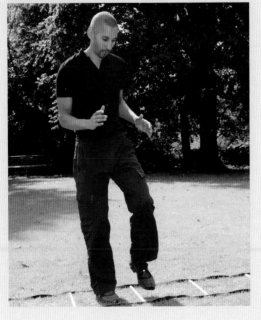

Starting position and action

- Stand behind a speed ladder with your feet together and knees slightly bent, leaning forward at the hips.
- Maintaining an upright but forward-leaning posture, step into the first rung of the speed ladder with your right leg.
- Then step immediately into the second rung with your left leg, followed immediately by stepping into the third rung with your right leg etc.
- Continue to step/run into each rung alternately with each leg through the ladder, ensuring you have fast footwork and are on the balls of your feet when you land.
- Complete one ladder then walk back and repeat 5–10 times.

Modifications

- This drill can be performed forwards/backwards or laterally (4.7b), pushing off your toes for each step.

Ex 4.8 Two feet in

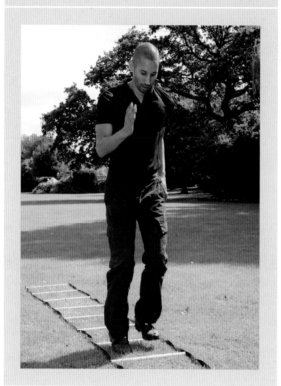

Modifications

- This drill can be performed backwards, following the similar stepping action but with backward pushing of the balls of your feet. Alternatively, it can be performed as a lateral drill, leading with the right leg travelling through the ladder to the right or leading with the left leg travelling through the ladder to the left.
- It is important to remain upright with a slight forward lean at your hips and pump the arms to assist your speed of leg movement while travelling through the ladder.

Starting position and action

- Stand behind a speed ladder as before, and this time step into the first rung of the ladder with your right leg, but follow immediately by stepping into the same rung with your left leg.
- Then step into the second rung with your right leg, followed by your left etc.
- Continue leading with your right leg and following with your left, maintaining your posture and staying on the balls of your feet with rapid steps, for the duration of the speed ladder.
- Complete the speed ladder and then walk back and repeat, this time leading with your left leg.
- Repeat a total of 6–10 times.

Ex 4.9 Two in, two out

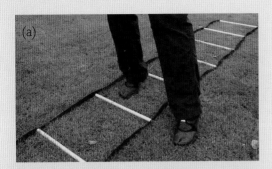

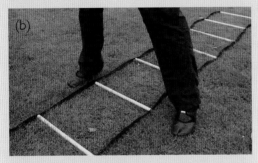

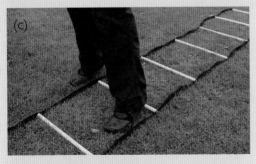

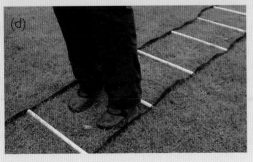

Starting position and action

- Stand in front of the speed ladder with feet hip-distance apart.
- Place your right foot in the first rung followed by your left foot also in the first rung, then place your right foot outside the ladder to the right and then your left foot outside the ladder to your left, in an in/in/out/out technique.
- Repeat this in/in/out/out technique for the second rung and progress through the ladder.

Modifications

- When repeating this drill, always try and change your lead leg, so that you are not favouring a specific movement pattern.
- Perform backwards, ensuring you are watching your stepping pattern and footwork together with the ladder rungs.
- Perform laterally, i.e. stand outside the ladder side-on to it and then, leading with your right leg at the bottom of the ladder with the ladder to your right, step into the first rung with your right foot and then your left, then step out with your right and then left foot.
- Continue to step in and out, but this time move on to the next rung, leading with your right leg, working your way along the ladder to your right in an in/in/out/out action.
- At the end, walk back and then stand on the other side and lead with your left leg as before.
- Repeat 4–10 times.

Ex 4.10 Mambo

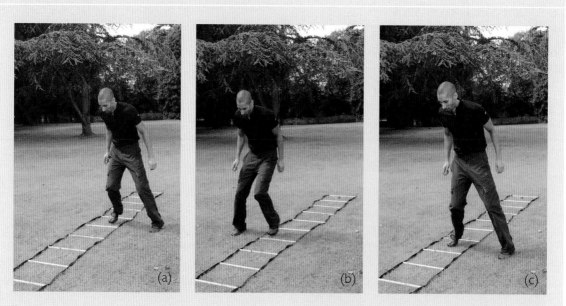

(a)   (b)   (c)

Starting position and action

- For this drill, the stepping action follows a 1/2/3 principle. In my experience, this drill is one of the hardest to master at speed.
- Stand in front of the speed ladder and step into the first rung of the ladder with your right foot.
- Then step into the first rung with your left foot.
- Step out of the ladder to your right with your right leg, but this time step with your left foot into the second rung of the speed ladder.
- Follow this by stepping into the second rung with your right leg and then step out of the ladder to your left, with your left leg.
- Repeat this in/in/out, in/in/out technique as you travel through the ladder.
- On reaching the end, walk back and repeat 5–10 times.

Modifications

- This drill can be performed backwards, but it is much harder.

TRAINING GUIDELINES AND EQUIPMENT

5

TRAINING GUIDELINES

In writing this book I wanted to provide a taste of activities and exercise options for all fitness levels and demonstrate specificity of training within certain disciplines, together with providing general outdoor exercise options for all enthusiasts. As such, this book does not focus on any specific training protocols, but is a collection of exercises and exercise options showing potential variations. There is no one definitive solution to any exercise programme, as everything can only ever be relative, subject to the desired goal, the equipment available, the time and intensity of training and also the ability of the participant in question.

For beginners embarking on a new training programme, it is important to try different workouts to see what is enjoyable and what you will maintain. For the more seasoned enthusiast, a structured programme would identify any muscular imbalances you might have and incorporates corrective exercises to strengthen weaker muscles while stretching tighter ones. This helps to redress the balance and '*synergy*' within your body. To reduce tightness in specific muscles you might want to try some of the foam-rolling exercises listed in the appendix. In this section you will find an explanation of foam-rolling techniques as well

as a guide to cool-down stretches to help stretch out muscles at the end of the workout.

For the sports enthusiast, interval training is fundamental in helping prepare your body and fitness levels for the demands of your sport. Your conditioning exercises should always have a functional element and involve core strength and endurance because without a strong core, your functional strength is compromised. As your core stabilisation improves you should incorporate more strength-related exercises, interspersed with advanced stabilisation exercises at moderate- to high-intensity intervals. Progress from here is to include more power-related exercises into your workouts. Remember that you should only apply these when a high level of core strength and motor-skill development relative to your training has been achieved. Everyone is different and what appears simplistic to one person might be difficult for another, so for a truly structured programme, always seek the advice of a reputable trainer at a local gym.

The following chapters provide examples of different interval workouts, such as a '*peripheral heart action*' circuit, which is simply an upper-body exercise followed by a lower-body exercise. This can be interspersed with an aerobic/anaerobic interval or it can be repeated. An alternate workout option is to perform a superset programme of opposing muscle groups interspersed with some cardio activity in an 'agonist/antagonist/cardiovascular (CV) workout. Giant sets' or mini circuits are another option, fused into a programme to combine three, four or five exercises performed within a circuit format before adding a cardio interval. It must be remembered that many functional exercises are dynamic in nature and consequently are challenging enough on their own, without the need to include any extra cardio.

Your workout length really depends on how much time you can make available. Workouts of twenty minutes performed twice a week will have some benefits as long as the intensity when training is sufficient. When starting out, if you are not used to a strength-training programme, choose 4–6 exercises that are simplistic in nature, yet work the full body. As you progress, incorporate a few more exercises ensuring you have a balance of major muscle groups: chest, shoulders, back, legs, arms and core, and that you vary the exercises and intensify the stabilisation element, such as by introducing a BOSU.

As a long-term plan you should train to include elements of strength and conditioning work that are functional in nature and that incorporate a variety of exercises, while always remembering to progress gradually. One of the biggest causes of injury while training is increasing your intensity or increasing the quantity of your workouts too quickly. With regards to the 'periodisation' or development of your programme, again it depends on the specificity of your goal, but as a rule, aerobic and endurance training will help prepare your baseline fitness for the more intense options of interval training. For the enthusiast, you could develop your programme by simply incorporating some of the more advanced exercises shown using the suspended body weight, ViPR and kettlebell equipment. But ultimately, as with all training, it comes down to your personal goals and motivation for training and, to a degree, the equipment and time you have available.

ABDOMINAL BRACING TECHNIQUES

Whenever you are required to lift, push, pull, throw, rotate or carry an object, demands are placed on the muscles used in the process. While the effort might be through your legs or arms, if your core muscles are not engaged effectively, then you risk causing injury. The important aspect is to remember to engage your core muscles by tensing or bracing them, according to the demands of the task. Bracing techniques really mean tensing the muscle isometrically (to minimise movement) and maintaining this tension throughout the movement as required.[20] However, whenever isometric tension is being applied, you should always maintain regular breathing, albeit compromised, and you should never hold your breath for more than a couple of seconds throughout the initial effort stage.

When performing movement and exercises using new portable equipment items, such as ViPRs and the TRX® Rip™ Trainer, you should be bracing your abdominals throughout, not just for each repetition, but from the moment you lift the ViPR from the floor or take hold of the TRX® Rip™ Trainer. It is likely that you will be performing quite dynamic movements throughout the exercise, so correct abdominal bracing or tensing is paramount throughout.

There are two main bracing techniques and it really comes down to the nature and intensity of movement performed, together with your own preference, to decide which to apply.

Abdominal bracing technique one

The first technique, often used when lifting heavier objects or when dynamic movement is applied, is to contract your core muscles simply by 'bracing' or tensing your core. No movement of the spine occurs and you should tense at about 40 per cent intensity, subject to your overload – tension that you can maintain for a short-lived duration but does not cause you to strain unduly. Consider if you were to pick up a heavy wheelbarrow by the handles. Your brain tells you that you need to protect your spine and have a solid foundation to work from, so prior to lifting you bend down, take hold of the handles and then 'brace' your core by contracting your abdominal muscles as you begin to lift. The trick is to keep this tension or bracing technique without holding your breath!

Abdominal bracing technique two

The second bracing technique is the more classic approach of drawing the naval inwards by contraction of your transverse abdominus and other core muscles, while simultaneously squeezing your pelvic floor muscles throughout.[21] Again, the focus of this contraction is to aim for about 40 per cent intensity, yet the nature of activity and potential forces to overcome might require greater contraction.

WEIGHT CONTROL

Weight loss is achieved by creating an energy imbalance, which forces your body to burn fat stores for energy. Your basal metabolic rate dictates the rate at which you digest, absorb and utilise the food you consume at rest. Whatever you do in addition to this creates your daily metabolism and dictates the total calorific expenditure for that day, whether this is working, shopping, cutting the grass or hiking for several miles. In simplistic terms, if you consume more calories than your total calorific expenditure, you put on weight or alternately, if you consume fewer calories or expend more than you normally consume, you lose weight.

Resistance training will enhance your metabolic rate, not only during the workout but also by training the muscles, which require energy to exist. The bigger and stronger the muscles, the more energy required to 'feed' them. However, unless weight training is fused with aerobic/anaerobic intervals or performed in such a way that your heart rate is elevated throughout (such as in circuit training) if weight loss is the goal, you should spend more time doing interval and/or aerobic training to help burn more calories. The more intense your workout, the greater the duration and the greater the frequency of workouts, the greater the amount of calories expended. There is no optimum workout plan – the one that works for you is the best plan, but, as a guide, eat carefully, train wisely and rest thoroughly.

EQUIPMENT

In Part Three, I have demonstrated a number of workouts in differing environments, starting with the most simplistic – walking – which requires no equipment other than a good pair of trainers and possibly a pedometer and/or heart-rate monitor. As you work through the various outdoor workouts, you will see I incorporate various pieces of equipment to supplement your workout and give greater variety in the exercises. Here is some of the equipment used in the exercises in this book:

Speed ladder

A speed ladder is simply a rope ladder with wooden or plastic rungs that is laid down on the ground, allowing you to run between the 'rungs'. It can vary in size, from 4m to 9m, and is available from most good sports shops or via the internet. It encourages improved motor-skill development through repeated running across the ladder with differing footwork drills. Because of the nature of the sprinting movements, you can also use this tool during interval training.

Hurdles

Hurdles come in different sizes and range from as low as 15cm to variable height hurdles, which can be set up to 1m in height. The lower ones can be used in speed and footwork drills or for low-level jumps and bounds, whereas the higher versions can be used for plyometric and jumping drills.

BOSU

BOSU stands for 'both sides utilised', which describes this tool's functionality perfectly. A BOSU is a semi-circular inflatable rubber ball that is flat on the other side. This means, depending upon which way up it is positioned, you can jump or step on to the BOSU and, due to its instability, it will cause you to have to stabilise your leg or whole body to remain balanced.

Many exercises can be performed on the BOSU and it is great when used with other resistance equipment such as dumbbells, ViPRs, medicine balls, etc.

Stability ball

Stability balls have been prominent in gyms since the late 1990s. They are used as a stabilisation bench to perform numerous exercises to challenge your deep-core muscles while sitting, lying or balancing on the stability ball. They are available in different sizes to suit the exerciser and usually range from 55cm to 75cm in diameter. Stability balls are unstable and so any movement performed on them requires a stabilisation element. As with much of the equipment mentioned, stability balls can be used in conjunction with many other resistance or stabilisation aids to challenge your fitness through various movements and drills.

Dumbbells

Dumbbells come in different weights, but it is important to have a sufficient weight for the exercise you are performing, as each muscle will have a different strength – a choice of two or three differing weights is usually sufficient. I would suggest using the heavier dumbbells for leg exercises, such as squats and lunges or even a chest press or single-arm row; medium resistance for shoulder press or biceps curls; and a lighter resistance for exercises such as triceps kickbacks or for core-stabilisation exercises.

Kettlebells

Kettlebells are essentially awkwardly shaped dumbbells with a handle. However, while a range of weights are now available, they are generally only available in heavier resistances than most dumbbells. You can perform most, if not all, dumbbell exercises with a kettlebell, but the design and nature of the kettlebell, with its handle 'outside' the main resistance, means that as you lift, it will respond differently to a dumbbell. As such, it is ideal for alternating swinging and combined movements to create total workouts.

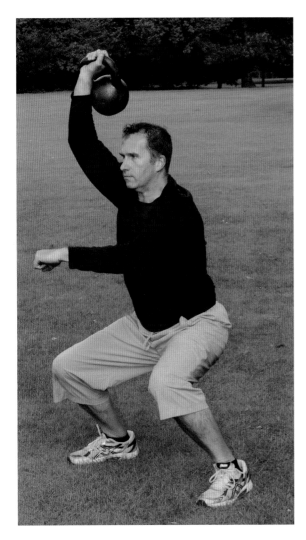

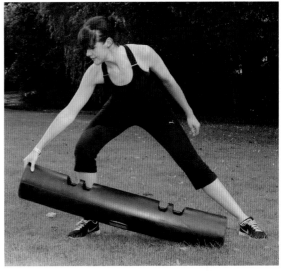

ViPRs

A ViPR is a heavy (4–20kg) cylindrical rubber tube with handles, which you can lift, carry, swing, drag and throw. ViPRs are unlike any previous training tool and an absolute must for all personal trainers because they encourage dynamic movement through all three planes of motion. All your muscles have to work together to overcome the resistance of the ViPR and the forces of its movement.

Tyres

Tyres are great in outdoor workouts because you don't have to worry about keeping them clean. You can use old car tyres, which you can drag behind you in sprint drills, carry, lift, throw or even hit with a sledgehammer! Should you be lucky enough to have a big garden, an old tractor tyre is a fantastic tool for lifting and flipping over a 10–20m distance, which creates an exhausting total-body workout. While spare car tyres are relatively portable in the boot of your car, tractor tyres offer less portability options.

Medicine ball

A medicine ball is a very versatile tool. It comes in various weights, usually 1–10kg, and is often made of plastic or leather. Again, depending upon the nature of the exercise, it might be worth having two sizes – one lighter (2–5kg) and one heavier (6–10kg), depending upon your fitness and strength. Unlike kettlebells or dumbbells, medicine balls lend themselves to power exercises, such as throwing and catching drills.

Punch bag

Punch bags are sometimes used in a bootcamp environment, where teams carry them across demanding terrain as part of an assault course. You can also carry lighter bags on your own. Again, their awkwardness makes the overall exercise harder, causing you to recruit more muscles in the process. They can be flipped, dragged, carried, lifted, pressed and (obviously) punched.

Powerbags

Powerbags usually come in 10kg, 15kg and 20kg resistances, but heavier ones can be obtained from specific equipment outlets or via the internet. Their advantage is that not only are they awkward to lift and carry, but they can be carried over a distance, dropped, picked up and thrown without damaging them.

Resistance tubes

A resistance tube is one of the cheapest and most user-friendly pieces of resistance kit available. They are available in graduated intensity (beginners, intermediate and advanced) and range in price from £4–15, but you can generally find a good one for under £10. You can stand on the tube and hold the grips so that when you perform an upper body exercise, the tube is stretched, which causes resistance. Alternatively, you can wrap the tube around a post or solid object so that you can perform a movement in any direction away from the post to create resistance as the tube is stretched.

Bungee cords

A bungee cord is useful when performing sprint drills, as it can provide a resistance to run against or can even assist your running, depending upon the direction and positioning. It can be positioned laterally to your movement so as to challenge core and leg muscles, which makes it useful in training for team and court sports.

Suspension Training® systems

Suspension Training® systems offers a fantastic way to get a total body workout. Unlike ViPRs or kettlebells, the suspension strap is completely portable and easily fits into a backpack. You secure the strap around a solid object or anchor point that will not move or break and that can comfortably take your bodyweight. From there, you can partially hang with your feet or hands on the floor (depending upon the exercise) and perform movements using your bodyweight as the resistance. Depending upon the extent of 'hang' or 'lean', you can decide upon the percentage of your bodyweight you are lifting and so control the intensity of the exercise. And it follows that as you begin to fatigue, you can reduce the intensity by adjusting your foot or even hand position. You only have to look at websites such as YouTube to see fitness enthusiasts and personal trainers performing a huge array of exercises using suspension straps, which will keep even the most die-hard enthusiasts challenged.

TRX® Rip™ Trainer

The TRX® Rip™ Trainer is a fantastic tool to really apply muscle integration while performing dynamic movements. It works a bit like a variable resistance tube on a stick, with one end of the TRX® Rip™ Trainer being secured, while you perform movements holding the lever bar. As the TRX® Rip™ Trainer is only secured to one end of the lever-bar element, you have to constantly brace your abdominals to perform any movement due to the asymmetric or one-sided pull effect it produces.

Cones

Cones are great to use as markers to run around or even to jump over, but in all honesty, for marking purposes you can use a T-shirt, twig or stone if need be.

Foam Roller

Foam rollers are used with self-myofascial release, a process that assists to 'roll out' tightness in muscles. This process is somewhat different from stretching in that it reduces tight spots or 'knots' in muscles, through pressure on the foam roller by placing it underneath the muscle as you sit, lay or apply your bodyweight.

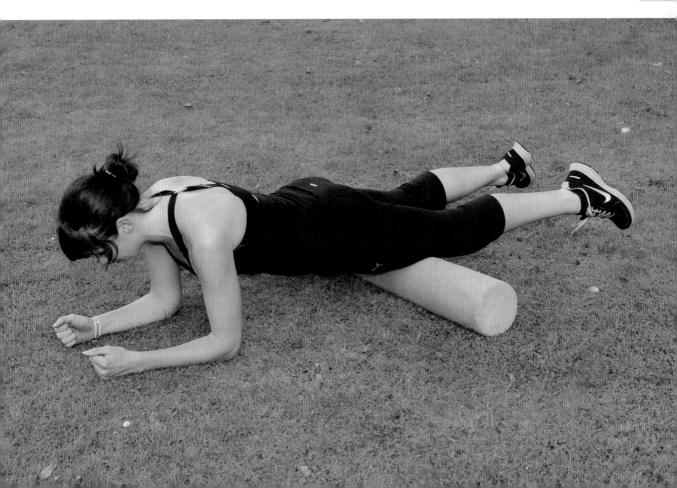

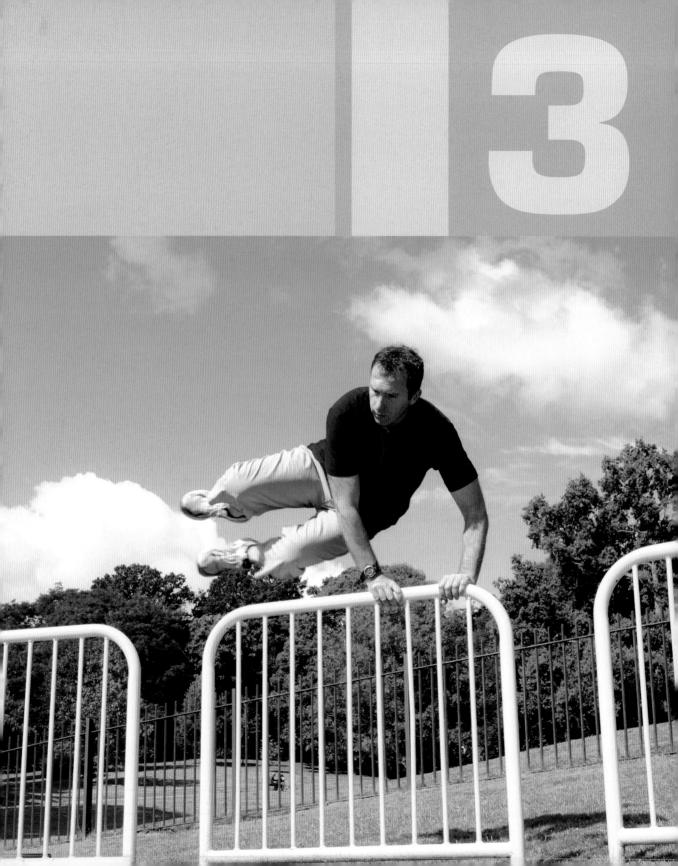

PART **THREE**

OUTDOOR
CONDITIONING
WORKOUTS

INTRODUCTION

Exercising outdoors can include many different activities, and whether you choose to get started with some gentle walking and build up from there, or you currently like running but don't want to spend money on a gym membership, maybe this section will tempt you into new outdoor workouts that can fit around your current fitness ideals. You might feel more comfortable within the surroundings of your own home and while a gym will certainly offer more options with regards to the fitness equipment available, air-conditioned studios and expert advice at hand, working out at a gym is not for everyone. In fact, you can achieve excellent results from simple exercises performed in your garden using minimal equipment that won't break the bank.

Part Three is where all the fun starts. You can choose from simple walking workouts or look to introduce jogging and running into your existing walks. You might be a recent mother who wants exercise options that enable you to have your new baby in tow. Maybe you are new to exercise and just want some ideas on getting started at home in the garden, or maybe you are a seasoned fitness enthusiast or personal trainer looking for some alternate ideas to spice up your current training programme.

Regardless of your goal, work through the next section chapter by chapter, to get a feel for the variety of exercises. This list is by no means exhaustive, nor have I tried to include every variation with every piece of fitness equipment; rather, I wanted to suggest possible variations that might be applicable in certain environments or that work best with certain resistance equipment. However, most exercises in each chapter are interchangeable. A push-up is a push-up, whether you do it on your knees in the garden, full-length off a breakwater, inverted with your feet raised off a park bench or while dangling between suspension straps. The choice really is down to you, your fitness level and your choice of equipment.

Remember to go gently at first if you are new to exercise and for the more advanced, try to master the technique at the lower intensity before performing the hardest variation. Always check with a doctor if you are embarking on exercises for the first time or if you are returning after a long break or as a result of an injury. More importantly, as you work your way through this next section, learn to listen to your body as it will usually tell you if it doesn't like a particular exercise.

As you progress through Part Three, you will see a range of fitness equipment you can utilise in an outdoor environment, yet by no means is all of it necessary for a complete total-body workout. So while you don't have to go out and buy equipment, I would strongly advise investing in a couple of items to add greater variety and resistance to your overall workout (*see* chapter 5 for examples). A stability ball or BOSU can be a useful aid to help challenge your core muscles as you perform various stabilisation bodyweight and resistance exercises. A simple resistance tube is both cost-effective and user-friendly, especially for new exercisers. Resistance tubes can be purchased in different resistance levels, suitable for beginners through to advanced, and are thus suitable for most exercises.

Should you want to invest further and as your interest in outdoor workouts develops, I would definitely recommend suspension straps, as this one piece of resistance kit, and the array of exercises that can be performed using it, will certainly keep you going as you progress. The versatility of suspension straps are that by simple adjustments in your stance and angle to the ground, your intensity can be greatly increased or decreased according to your body position.

Whether you are interested in walk/run plans and you simply want to add a few bodyweight exercises to your workout, or you like the idea of working out at home, at the beach or park, or even if you decide to sign up to a professional bootcamp, Part Three will offer plenty of ideas to help you on your way.

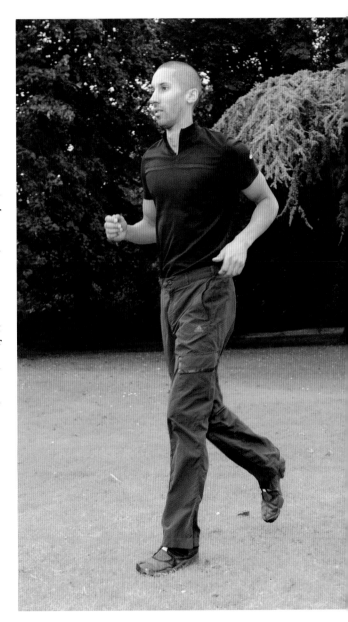

WALKING AND RUNNING

FITNESS WALKING

Walking is undoubtedly the most accessible form of exercise and it can be simply walking around your local park or a day or two on a hiking or back-packing trip. (For the latter, of course, you really need to know where you are going, wear suitable clothing and have sufficient equipment and/or subsistence to make the event safe and enjoyable.) For the purposes of this book, I want to promote the benefits of walking.

When you look to progress your fitness walking, it is important to know your limits. Maybe you are comfortable with a simple stroll around the block or a visit to the park. Perhaps you can walk for 5km or you think nothing of a weekend stroll lasting 2–3 hours. The important thing is that you start with what you *can* do and progress from there, safely and effectively, by increasing a combination of frequency, intensity and duration.

The benefits of regular walking include:

- a reduction in blood pressure;
- improved cholesterol levels;
- improved muscle tone in the legs;
- an increase in bone density due to the low impact movement; and

- accessibility: anyone can do it, whatever fitness level or age. You simply open your front door and off you go.

WALKING TECHNIQUE

When walking, try to avoid looking down and aim to keep looking forwards towards the horizon. Keep your arms bent at 90 degrees, but make sure you keep your shoulders relaxed – don't tense them up. Swing your arms as you walk, moving them forcefully forwards and back to assist your pace, but try not to over-exaggerate the arm action – just walk a little faster and pump your arms to help speed up your legs.

For race walking, the technique is completely different. While the principle is that you walk as fast as you can, the technique relies on dynamic and powerful movements. Race walking utilises technical foot strikes and hip rotations to assist the movement and allow for greater speed. The technicalities of race walking go beyond the scope of this book, and should you wish to pursue the activity we recommend researching appropriate resource material for a fuller explanation of techniques and training.

Before pursuing walking as a fitness option, you should invest in a good pair of trainers. While running shoes are not always the best option, since the heel cushioning can often be too great, as long as you have comfortable shoes that give you support and a degree of cushioning, then off you go. Flip-flops are definitely not suitable. If your longer-term goals are rambling and hiking in the countryside, you might want to seek out specific walking shoes with greater ankle stability but to begin with, a good pair of trainers will usually suffice.

As for the distance and intensity of your walk, the decision is up to you. Initially you should focus on what is manageable, such as a walk around the block, and build up to a couple of miles or so. When you are comfortable fitness walking for 30–45 minutes or longer, why not consider a change of scenery and introduce walks in a park or the countryside and, if you like it, consider doing a half-day ramble or even a hike. Alternatively, if your fitness has improved and you wanted to try the occasional jog, even for 50 metres, this could be the start of a walk/run plan as shown on page 55. Wherever your fitness walking takes you, enjoy it, as there is no simpler way of getting active in the outdoors.

JOGGING

There is one thing that cannot be denied when considering jogging as both a fitness and weight-loss tool and that is its accessibility and cost-effectiveness – all that it requires is a good pair or trainers and somewhere safe to jog.

Human beings are very capable of running and we have all jogged at one stage in our lives, whether for a bus, in the playground evading capture in a game of tag, or getting to a parking meter before the inspector sees that you are beyond your allocated time.

Yet all too often clients come to me and say they can't run. For those who are grossly overweight or have specific injuries, running could be a foolish choice, I agree; I personally don't advise someone of average build who is over 100kg to take up jogging, unless they are a competitive athlete and have suitable conditioning, as the risk of injury due to impact forces to ankles, hips, knees, shins and calves probably outweighs the potential fitness benefits. However, if weight loss and improved fitness is the long-term goal, and if you can walk for over 30 minutes at a good speed and you are not excessively overweight, then jogging is always an option.

EMBARKING ON A JOGGING PROGRAMME

Before starting any running programme, the first and most important thing you will need is a good pair of trainers. If you are just starting out you shouldn't need to spend more than £50 on a quality pair. Seek advice from a reputable sports store on the most suitable shoe for your running style. Also, some shoes have more cushioning and are suitable for the heavier runner, while others have greater stability and lateral support for those who require ankle support.

With any fitness programme, the important element is that it develops to challenge your ability without causing injuries through adding intensity, distance or volume too quickly. There is no need for the initial distance to be excessively high – as part of a fitness and weight-loss programme for the unfit, total distances and running distance can begin at a relatively low level, but should look to increase gradually according to your goals. Therefore, before you jump straight into running, you should aim to build up slowly with a walk/run programme (walking, then running, then walking, etc.), which will gradually increase your overall jog/run time over a period of weeks.

A walk/jog programme might start with you walking the distance between two lampposts and then jogging the distance between the next two lampposts, according to your base fitness level. Repeat this walk/jog 10–20 times so that you might have run up to 20 'double lamppost lengths' of 30–40m (thus a total distance of half a kilometre up to three-quarters of a kilometre with perhaps a total walking distance of similar or more). This would mean a total distance covered of between 1km and 2km. If you are on a treadmill, you might aim for a 45–90-second jog followed by a 30–60-second walk. A simple timing period of one minute jogging followed by one minute walking is easy to remember and follow, repeating these intervals for 10–20 minutes.

The next step is to focus on your total specific jog/run length, i.e. the length of time you can maintain your jog/run without stopping or reducing to a walk. Remember though: if weight loss is your goal, for optimum calorie expenditure, the greater the duration and the higher the intensity, the greater amount of calories burned. Regardless of fitness, you should always respect the run and how your body responds to it. (For more walk/run plans see pages 55–56).

JOGGING WARM UP

You should always warm up relative to the intensity of your run. If you intend a high-level sprint session then your warm-up drills will need to be very specific and involve varying graduations of sprinting in the session. However, for a basic jog or run, the important factor is that the muscles are warm and the joints mobilised.

A basic warm-up for a moderate jogging/running session should include the principles below.

- Start with general mobilisation of the ankle (ankle circles) and then bend the knees, lifting them to waist height a few times.
- Rotate gently through the trunk while dynamically loosening the arms and shoulders with an exaggerated running action, perhaps by slowly bringing the knees up to touch alternate elbows.
- Then start by walking, exaggerating the heel-toe action, by exaggerating the heel strike and rolling through to push off your toes. Then follow by a few seconds of walking on tiptoe and then a few seconds walking on your heels. Continue this for a minute or so.
- Then increase your walking pace over a couple of minutes and mix in some gentle jogging and power-walking and finally graduate towards your normal jogging/running speed.

JOGGING/RUNNING TECHNIQUE

Depending on your speed and the distance you intend to jog, your arm position should be relaxed and comfortable and you should ideally keep your wrists approximately level with your belly button. Try not to grip too tightly with your fist as this can cause tension in your forearms, arms and possibly shoulders over a period of time. Your body position should be upright but not rigid, which will help to reduce tension in the shoulders. You should also be thinking about your landing action with special attention to your foot strike (i.e. where and how your foot hits the ground). Ideally you should be following a heel-toe running action so that your body weight and landing forces are distributed through the foot, landing on your heel and rolling through your foot to push off your toes. This helps to perpetuate the running action. A way to gauge this is to try and listen to the sound when your foot strikes the ground. Ideally there should be minimal sound when your foot hits the floor, which means that the cushioning effect is maximised.

Interval sessions

If you are new to running, the most common mistake is to start too quickly – in other words, you begin at an intensity that you cannot sustain. The result is that after 400–800m you will find your heart in your mouth, your head pounding and every bodily function screaming at you to stop. The solution is to set yourself realistic goals and don't expect too much too quickly – listen to your body.

For those runners who are looking to improve their times, one method might be through interval sessions on certain run days. This will assist both your leg speed and also improve your overall fitness. Interval sessions can include hill work and/or speed variations and an example of what you might include in a sprint training interval session is shown below in table 6.1.

The sprint training intervals can be included in a 'fartlek', or 'speed play', running session, but usually in a less structured manner. For example, you could incorporate repeatedly attacking a hill route into your run, using lampposts as markers to add repeated sprints or even high-knee

Table 6.1	Example interval sessions
Reps/distance	**Session**
3–5 x 300–400m	Uphill running at a gradient of 3–5% at 80% intensity (very high effort level). Allow recovery by walking or jogging back to start.
4–6 x 100–150m	Uphill running at a gradient of 15–20% at 90% effort (near maximal effort). Return to start by walking back down.
6 x 60m sprints	Sprint 60m at 90–100% effort level. Walk or slow jog back to the start, allowing heart rate to return to a comfortable level.
5 x 30–40m bounding	Take exaggerated running leaps (bounding – see Ex 8.32, p. 109), aiming to minimise the number of strides over a set distance.
8 x 25m sprints	Sprint 25m at 100% effort (maximum speed or effort level), aiming to achieve maximum acceleration and speed, walk back for recovery.
10 x 10–15m	From a moving start, sprint 10–15m and then jog for 20m and continue in the same direction, or around a track/field.
8 x 50–80m	Tyre pulls using a harness, or use a bungee cord across a flat or slightly inclined field.

skipping and other footwork drills (*see* chapters 3 and 4).

Hill running

When running up a hill your body position should have a slightly greater forward lean. You will need to lift your knees higher and try and 'attack' the hill/gradient, so that you drive harder with your legs and arms for the duration of the hill. When running down a hill, depending on the gradient, you should try not to 'brake' with your legs but rather allow the hill to dictate your leg action and

leg speed. This will take a few weeks to master but the important aspect is to remain in control of the movement while running at a faster speed than normal.

Beginners' walk/run programme

Table 6.2 shows a simple walk/run plan in which you have three workouts per week. Each workout includes the total amount of time for the workout and the cumulative time you should aim to run for, not necessarily constantly but in 1/2/3/4/5 minute intervals interspersed with 1–2 minutes of walking. As you progress, simply extend the running times and minimise the walking times.

Marathon

Should your interest or motivation for running take hold, you might want to attempt greater distances than within the beginners guide. You might want to attempt a 10km distance, compete in a half marathon or even work your way up to running a full marathon. Providing you are able to complete week 6 from table 6.2 and can run for 3–5 miles then there is absolutely no reason you could not train for a full marathon, following the simplistic training guide in table 6.3. The important element is to increase your mileage gradually to avoid unnecessary injuries.

When attempting a marathon for the first time, without a specific time goal, the emphasis is to generate 'time on your feet' by increasing total mileage gradually, while increasing your long steady run gradually as well. Other runs should be of medium duration but perhaps at a higher intensity, with shorter runs to include speed work, hill training and threshold training to improve your fitness level.

Running tips

Do:

- wear a good pair of running shoes;
- warm up by graduating your intensity of walking/running;
- keep a relaxed arm movement to reduce shoulder stress;
- get into a natural breathing rhythm;
- wear comfortable clothing that allows your skin to breathe;
- always keep hydrated during and after your run;
- as you finish your run, always remember to cool down and stretch, paying particular attention to your calf muscles, hamstrings and quad muscles.

Don't:

- exaggerate your running action – keep the movement natural;
- push too hard, too soon;
- try to keep up with the person that passes you in the park.

Table 6.2	Beginners' walk/run programme					
Week	Workout 1		Workout 2		Workout 3	
	Total time (mins)	Run time (mins)	Total time (mins)	Run time (mins)	Total time (mins)	Run time (mins)
1	5–10	3–5	7–12	4–7	8–15	5–9
2	10–15	7–10	12–16	8–12	13–18	9–14
3	15–20	10–15	17–22	12–16	18–25	13–17
5	20–25	15–20	22–28	17–23	23–30	18–24
5	25–30	20–25	27–33	22–28	28–35	23–30
6	30–40	25–35	35–45	28–40	40–50	35–45

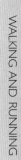

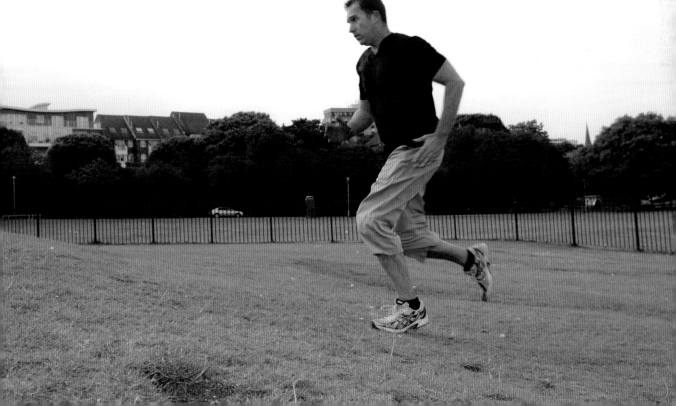

| Table 6.3 | 15-week marathon training guide |

Week	Training (miles)/rest days						
	Days of the week						
	1	2	3	4	5	6	7
1	1–3 S	Rest	2–3	Rest	1–2 H	Light CV	Rest
2	4–5 S	Rest	2–3 *	Rest	2–4 H	Rest	1–2 Hills
3	5–6 S	Rest	3–4	Rest	2–4 H	1–3 *	Rest
4	6–7 S	Rest	2–4 *	Rest	2–5 H	1–3 Hills	Rest
5	8–9 S	Rest	4–5	CV – 20	2–3 H	Rest	Rest
6	10–12 S	Rest	2–4 *	Rest	3–5 H	1–3 Hills	Rest
7	11–14 S	Rest	4–6	Rest	4–6 H	2–3 *	Light CV
8	12–15 S	Rest/light CV	5–6	Rest	3–5 *	2–3 Hills	Light CV
9	13–16 S	Rest/light CV	2–5 *	CV – 20	Rest	2–4 Hills	Rest
10	15–17 S	Rest/light CV	2–5 *	CV – 30	6–8	3–4 Hills	Rest
11	18–20 S	Rest/light CV	3–5*	CV – 45	7–9	2–4 *	Light CV
12	19–22 S	Rest/light CV	4–6	CV – 30	8–10	Light CV	Rest
13	14–16 S	Rest/light CV	3–5	Rest	5–8 H	Light CV	Rest
14	7–10 S	Rest	3–5	Rest	2–4	Rest	1–2
15	Marathon	Rest/light CV	Rest	1–3	Rest	CV 20–30	3–5

Key

- **S** Steady run
- ***** Interval session – speed work or aerobic threshold training
- **H** Hard run – run at faster pace than is comfortable
- **Hills** Hill-training intervals
- **Light CV** 20–30 minutes' cardio – non/low impact
- **CV** 20–45 minutes cardio

GARDEN
WORKOUT

7

If exercising at home makes sense to you, then the next chapter will provide some exercise ideas that might appeal. The garden workout gives examples of exercises that can be realistically achieved in most small to medium gardens, and which don't require excessive space or lots of equipment. In fact, I have based them specifically on exercises that I have performed with clients when working as a freelance personal trainer in their homes or gardens. Even if you only have a small backyard, many of the drills can be adapted and performed without too much compromise.

I have grouped the exercises together to cover cardio and agility drills, followed by those that lend themselves to specific muscle groups. Some of the exercises cover multiple muscle groups and

can be considered to be total-body exercises. In this instance, I have identified the major muscle group targeted in the exercise and have included it in the relevant section. Towards the end of the chapter there are several suggested workout plans and you will also find several challenging exercises, which provide greater options for the relatively fit and accomplished home exerciser. But, as with all exercise handbooks, this list is not exhaustive and many of the exercises from future chapters could be substituted or included in your workout at home.

You might feel uncomfortable performing some of the exercises in this chapter; if so, simply choose another. Remember to follow the warm-up guidelines from chapter 3 before attempting any of the exercises.

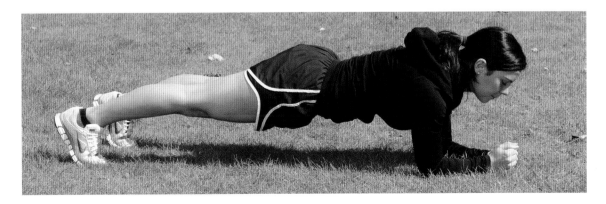

CARDIO AND AGILITY DRILLS

Ex 7.1 Jumping jacks

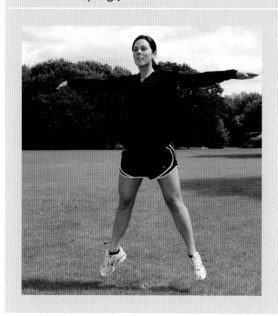

Ex 7.2 Air jacks/stars

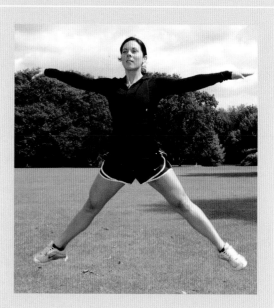

Starting position and action

- This is a classic aerobic exercise requiring no equipment.
- Stand with feet together, knees slightly bent and arms by your side.
- Keeping your abdominals braced, push off your legs to launch yourself into the air so that you land with feet in a wide stance.
- As your legs separate out to the side, also abduct your arms, bringing them to a horizontal position upon landing.
- From this 'star' landing position, bend both legs ready to jump back into the feet-together position as your arms return back your sides.
- Repeat this 'jumping jack' technique for 20–30 repetitions.

Starting position and action

- This is a more advanced version of the jumping jack as it requires a greater 'push off' into the air, thus requiring greater effort.
- Start as before with feet together and knees slightly bent, with your arms by your side.
- Squat down partially before pushing off with force through your legs and glutes to launch yourself into the air. This time as you jump, abduct your arms and legs into a 'star' position before returning them back to the start position as you return to the ground.
- Bend your knees as you land with your feet together to 'cushion' your landing on each jump.
- Push off your legs jumping up and into a star position again before landing with feet together as before. Repeat for 20–30 repetitions.

Ex 7.3 Kangaroos

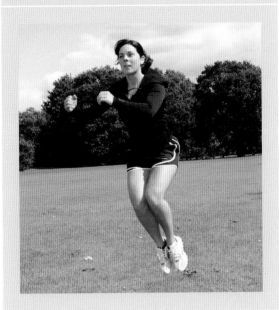

Starting position and action

- Begin with your feet together and your knees slightly bent, with arms by your sides.
- Squat down slightly to add power to your jump and then swing your arms forwards and upwards, keeping them slightly bent to assist your jump as you leap diagonally to your right.
- As you land, keeping your knees together and bending your knees to absorb your landing forces, push off through your legs, this time jumping to your left.
- Repeat these 'zigzag' jumps, keeping your feet and knees together as you repeatedly jump down the garden for 15–20m.
- Aim to jump as far as you can with each jump, cushioning your landing each time by partially squatting down before jumping back up.

Ex 7.4 Squat thrusts

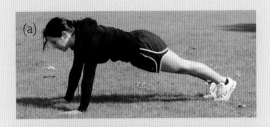
(a)

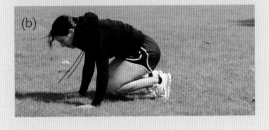
(b)

Starting position and action

- Start in a prone position on your hands and feet with your hands shoulder-width apart and your knees bent, with feet separated and approximately under your hips.
- Taking your weight on to your arms, brace your abdominals and drive both feet back into an extended position, to land with both feet together at the same time ensuring you are not dropping your hips but keeping your pelvis and back stabilised.
- From the extended position, lean into your arms to take more of your bodyweight again as you push off your toes and drive your knees in towards your chest into the start position.
- Repeat this for 30–50 repetitions.

Modifications

- When in the extended position, perform a push-up before returning to the start position in the way described above.

EXERCISES FOR THE CORE

Ex 7.5 Abdominal bridges/planks*

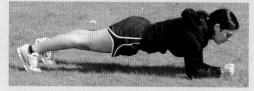

*Image shows modification

Starting position and action
- Kneel down on the floor and lean forwards so that your bodyweight is supported on your forearms and shoulders.
- Brace your abdominals, maintaining spinal alignment, and ensure that your hips do not drop below 15cm from the floor.
- Hold position for 20–45 seconds and then sit back on your knees to recover.
- After a 10–15-second rest, repeat the exercise for 3–5 bracing positions or 'bridges'.

Modifications
- To increase the intensity, straighten your legs one at a time so that your weight balances on your toes.
- Maintain this position for 20–60 seconds according to your core endurance and repeat as before 2–3 times.
- When this becomes less challenging, try raising one foot slightly off the floor for half of the time you intend to hold the bridge for, lowering and raising the other foot for the remainder.
- (*see* Ex 7.8, p. 62).

Ex 7.6 Abdominal curls on stability ball*

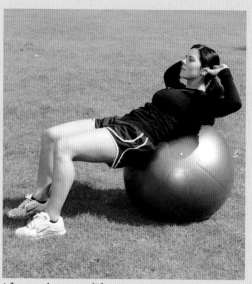

*Image shows modification

Starting position and action
- Lie over a stability ball face up with your arms across your chest, hands touching opposite shoulders.
- Position yourself on the stability ball with your lower and mid-back touching the ball with your knees bent and your feet hip-distance apart on the floor.
- Brace your abdominals initially to help stabilise yourself and then slowly curl up, contracting your abdominals to lift your mid-back away from the ball as your chest lifts upwards, curling towards your hips.
- Curl up until your torso is fully flexed but your hips remain in the start position with your lower back still on the stability ball.
- Hold this position briefly before lowering back to the start position.
- Do 12–20 repetitions.

Modifications

- To intensify this exercise you can take your hands behind your head to increase the level length.
- Alternatively, hold on to a light medicine ball or dumbbell, or even secure a resistance tube to a door or post behind you and curl against the resistance of the tube.
- To reduce the intensity, place your hands on your thighs.
- To increase the stabilisation requirement, place your feet together or even raise one foot off the floor.

Ex 7.7 Supermans

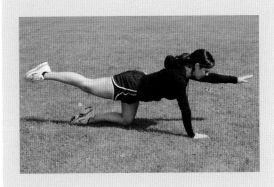

Starting position and action

- Position yourself on your hands and knees, with your hands under your shoulders.
- Brace your abdominals, maintaining spinal alignment, and slowly raise your left arm in front of you at a 45-degree angle to the spine, keeping your thumb pointing upwards.
- Simultaneously extend your right leg behind you while maintaining correct abdominal tension and spinal alignment, aiming to get the raised arm and leg parallel to the floor.
- Hold this extended position for 5–10 seconds and then slowly return to the start position, before repeating with the opposite arm and leg.

Modifications

- To intensify the stabilisation demands of this drill, try performing the movement on a BOSU, or for a real challenge, on a stability ball.

Ex 7.8 Dynamic planks

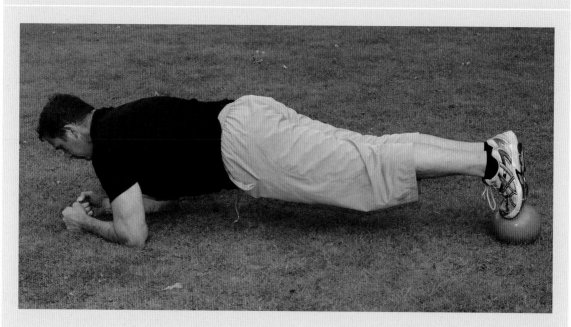

Starting position and action

- Lie face down on the floor with your elbows and forearms underneath your chest.
- Lift your hips up and, bracing your abdominals, place your feet (one at a time) on a medicine ball.
- Keep your spine in neutral and your legs straight, with your bodyweight being supported through your elbows and forearms and your feet on the ball.
- Hold this position for 30 seconds–1 minute before lowering your knees to the floor and taking your feet off the medicine ball to recover.
- Repeat the plank position for 2–5 repetitions.

Modifications

- To reduce the intensity, place your feet on a BOSU (flat side down) or even a cushion.

- An alternate body position is to support yourself on your hands in a straight arm position with hands shoulder-width apart and your body in neutral alignment.
- To challenge yourself even further, hold on to the sides of a BOSU with your hands in a push-up position and with both feet on the medicine ball. In this position you could add a push-up to the exercise, lowering your chest towards the BOSU before extending your arms back to the start position.
- To increase the stabilisation effect further, try having only one foot on the ball when you are in the plank position and change your balancing foot every 10 seconds, holding the other leg in the air 15–30cm away.

Ex 7.9 Stability ball roll-ins

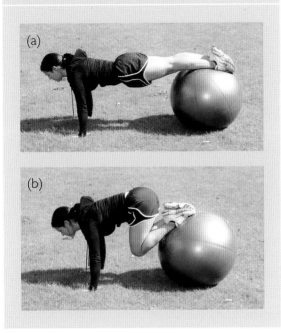

(a)

(b)

Ex 7.10 Stability ball lying torso rotations

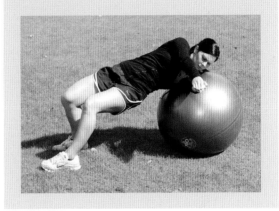

Starting position and action

- Begin with your hands on the floor underneath your shoulders and the stability ball near your feet.
- Place your legs (one at a time) on top of the stability ball so that your shins are in contact with the ball.
- Maintaining abdominal tension, bend both your knees, lifting your hips and drawing your knees towards your chest so that with your feet/shins on the stability ball, the ball rolls towards you underneath your hips.
- Pause briefly before extending your legs to roll the ball back to the start position.
- Do 10–15 complete repetitions.

Starting position and action

- Lie face up on a stability ball with your arms extended overhead and your shoulders and upper back in contact with the ball.
- Clasp your hands together and push your hips upwards to keep your torso and thighs parallel to the floor with your feet hip-distance apart.
- Maintain abdominal tension and roll over to your right, coming up on to your right shoulder by twisting through your torso so that your arms are pointing to your right and are almost parallel to the floor.
- Then rotate to your left, maintaining core tension throughout and repeat, this time coming up on to your left shoulder and alternating to your right and left for 20–30 repetitions.

Modification

- To increase the stabilisation demands, bring your feet closer together.

Ex 7.11 Stability ball roll-outs

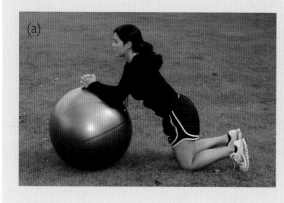 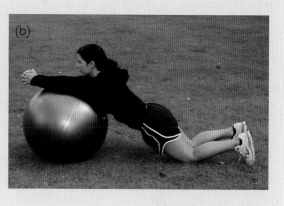

Starting position and action

- Kneel behind a stability ball and place your clasped hands together on top of the ball, in front of you.
- Roll the ball away slightly, with your abdominals braced as you begin to lean on to the ball, taking your weight through your arms, keeping the ball under your forearms and elbows.
- Lean forwards over the ball as far as you can comfortably while on your knees. Pause briefly, keeping your abdominals braced, before rolling the ball back into the starting kneeling position.
- Repeat this rolling-out-and-in movement yet adjust the starting position according to the difficulty level and your own ability; the further you place your hands and roll the ball away from your body as you lean forwards the greater the resistance.
- Do 10–12 repetitions.

Modifications

- To really challenge your core muscles, this exercise can be performed from a standing position or you can begin from a kneeling position, but as the ball is rolled away from your torso, with your forearms on top of the ball, you can extend your legs to come up on to your feet.
- This extra resistance will greatly increase the intensity of the exercise and so maintaining correct alignment by bracing your abdominals throughout is very important.

Ex 7.12 Stability ball kneeling balance

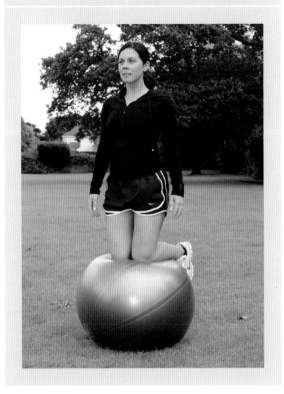

- Very carefully, maintaining abdominal tension, take your hands off the wall to challenge your balance without assistance.
- Hold this balance for periods of 5–15 seconds initially, building up to 45 seconds or even 1 minute.

Modifications
- When you can maintain a relatively stable kneeling position on the ball, if you have a partner to pass you dumbbells, many resistance exercises can be attempted while kneeling on the stability ball.
- In addition, a number of medicine ball exercises including throwing and catching techniques will be much harder if performed in a kneeling position while on the stability ball.

Starting position and action
- Start near a wall, which will help you to get on to the ball.
- Hold the wall and place your right knee and shin on to the ball.
- Keeping your balance by holding the wall, place your left leg on to the ball so that you are kneeling with the ball under your shins, sitting back on your heels.
- In this position, brace your abdominals to help stabilise yourself and lift yourself up so that your spine and hips are in neutral, still holding on to the wall.

Ex 7.13 Stability ball lateral crunches

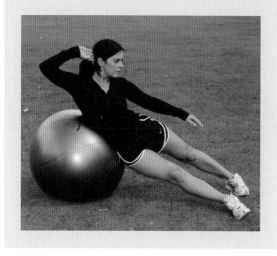

Ex 7.14 Super-slow bicycles

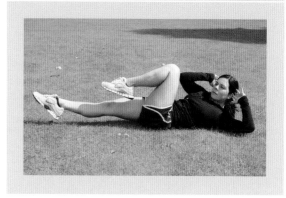

Starting position and action

- Lie across the stability ball on your right side, with your right arm over the ball and your feet separated and on the floor.
- Squeeze your oblique muscles, flexing at the waist, to lift your torso off the ball.
- Reach across your left hip with your left hand reaching down your thigh.
- Pause briefly at the top position before lowering back slowly across the ball.
- Do 15–20 repetitions.

Starting position and action

- Lie down on the floor facing upwards with your hands behind your head.
- Partially contract your abdominals to lift your shoulders and upper back off the floor.
- Then lift your left knee towards your chest and extend your right leg out at about 45 degrees.
- Brace your abdominals and rotate your torso slightly to bring your right elbow and shoulder towards your left knee.
- Hold this position briefly before changing your leg position and rotating slightly to your right so that your right knee is over your chest and you have curled your left elbow towards it, with your left leg extended.
- You should keep this movement slow over a 2–3 second count and aim for 15–30 repetitions in total.

Ex 7.15 Commando crawls

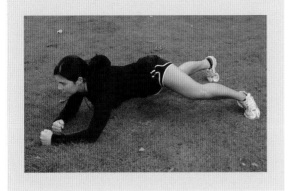

EXERCISES FOR THE CHEST

Ex 7.16 Push-ups on your knees

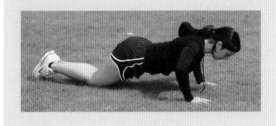

Starting position and action

- Begin in a prone position, yet with your weight supported on your elbows, lying on your tummy, hips and thighs.
- Crawl yourself forwards on your arms and forearms, pushing off your legs in a 'lizard-like' fashion, to crawl forwards over a distance of 10–20m.

Starting position and action

- Begin on your knees with your hands on the floor, slightly wider than shoulder-width apart, supporting your bodyweight.
- Keeping your body in alignment and abdominals braced, slowly bend your arms to lower to the floor, keeping your head in neutral.
- As you reach the floor, maintaining your abdominal tension, push against the floor to lift back to the start position.
- Do 10–20 repetitions, keeping the movement smooth and controlled.

Modifications

- When you can comfortably achieve over 20 repetitions, move on to a full-length position.
- Keep your body straight but come up on to your feet, straightening your legs and maintaining abdominal tension. Aim for 1–10 repetitions, initially.
- When you can't achieve another full-length repetition lower your knees to the floor and try another 5–10 repetitions.

Ex 7.17 Push-ups with rotation

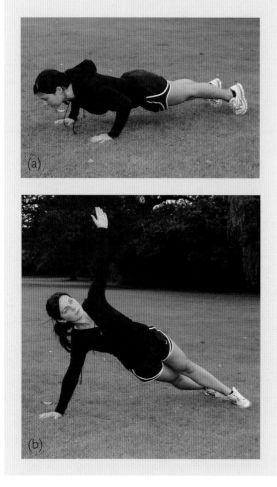

(a)

(b)

Starting position and action

- Begin in a push-up position, face down with hands shoulder-width apart and arms extended under your shoulders and your legs outstretched behind you.
- Maintain abdominal tension throughout this exercise and slowly bend your arms to lower yourself to the floor, bringing your chest 15cm from the floor (Ex 7.17a).

- Then extend your arms, working your chest, shoulders and triceps to push yourself back toward the start position.
- As your arms near a straight position, shift your weight on to your right arm and toes and rotate your torso to the left while lifting your left arm upwards to point towards the ceiling.
- This rotation will 'open up' this push position so that you are balanced on your right hand and toes (Ex 7.17b).
- Hold this position briefly before rotating back and placing your left hand on the floor under your left shoulder, then bend both arms as before to lower your chest and torso to the floor.
- Push up again, this time taking your weight on to your left hand and rotating to your right, to lift your right arm in the air, pausing briefly before rotating back and lowering to the floor with both arms.
- In order to lift your hand off the floor, you have to apply greater force to the pushing aspect of the push-up and shift your weight slightly to one side.

Modification

- This exercise can be performed with your knees on the floor to reduce the intensity, yet still ensure you maintain abdominal bracing throughout. The reduced lever-effect of being on your knees will, however, compromise your rotation ability so be careful not to flex unnecessarily at your hips.

Ex 7.18 Single-arm stability ball chest presses

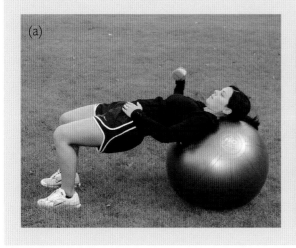

Starting position and action

- Lie back over a stability ball face up and lift your hips so that your head, neck and shoulders are in contact with the stability ball.
- Hold a dumbbell in your right hand by your chest, with your right arm bent and elbow below the dumbbell.
- Brace your abdominals and press the dumbbell upwards, over your chest, keeping your left hand loosely resting on your abdomen.
- At the top position, pause briefly before slowly lowering the dumbbell back to your chest.
- Ensure when you press the dumbbell you do not twist or 'squirm' to assist the movement.
- Do 10–15 repetitions before changing hands and repeating with your left hand.
- For added stability, begin with your feet wide and as your ability improves, narrow your foot placement until feet are hip-distance apart or even together.

Modifications

- If this proves too challenging, place a dumbbell in each hand to balance out the resistance and thus make the stabilisation slightly easier.
- Alternatively, try the single-arm chest press from a bench, if available, or even the floor.
- To increase the stabilisation further, take one leg off the floor (opposite to the hand holding the dumbbell).

Ex 7.19 Stability ball push-ups

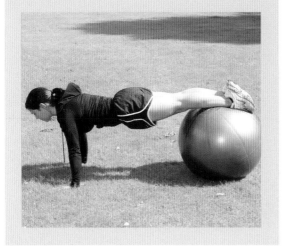

EXERCISES FOR THE BACK

Ex 7.20 Stability ball cobras

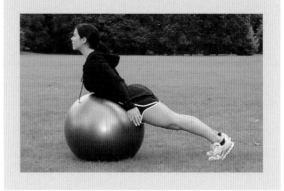

Starting position and action

- Lie over the stability ball in a prone position, with your hips and upper thighs on the ball and your hands on the floor in front of you.
- Place your hands slightly wider than shoulder-width apart in a push-up position.
- Brace your abdominals and keep your body rigid throughout the movement.
- Bend your arms to lower your chest to the floor, keeping your abdominals braced.
- As your chin or chest nears the floor, push down with your arms to lift yourself back to the start position.
- Exhale as you push yourself back to the starting position and repeat 10–15 times.

Modification

- When you can comfortably perform 15–20 repetitions, position the stability ball further down your legs so that it lies under your (i) knees, (ii) shins (iii) ankles or (iv) toes.

Starting position and action

- Kneel behind the stability ball and lie over it, face down with your torso and hips resting on the ball, and then extend your legs behind you with your feet hip-distance apart and your arms in front of you with your hands together.
- With your abdominals braced, extend your back to lift your chest off the ball, keeping your head in neutral alignment.
- As you lift up, separate your arms and keeping your thumbs up, retract your shoulder blades to bring your arms into a lowered crucifix position.
- Pause briefly in this raised position, squeezing your shoulder blades together and then return to the start position slowly.
- Repeat 8–12 times.

Modifications

- To increase intensity, bring your feet together.
- To add stability, place your feet wider apart.

Ex 7.21 Stability ball back extensions *

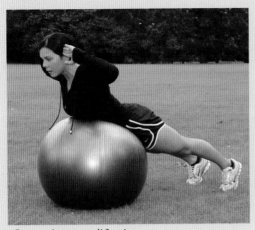

* Image shows modification

Starting position and action

- Kneel behind the stability ball and lie over it, face down with your torso and hips resting on the ball, and then extend your legs behind you with your feet hip-distance apart and your arms by your sides.
- With your abdominals braced, extend your back to lift your chest off the ball, keeping your head in neutral alignment.
- Rise up to bring your spine into a partially hyper-extended position, pausing briefly, ensuring you are not trying to lift too far, before slowly lowering your chest back over the stability ball.
- Repeat 8–12 times, keeping the movement slow and controlled.

Modification

- To increase the intensity bring your hands by your head or even extend your arms out in front of you, in line with your torso, thus increasing the level length and intensifying the movement further.

Ex 7.22 Supine shoulder retractions

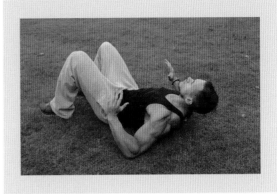

Starting position and action

- Begin lying on the floor in a supine position with your arms across your chest and knees bent with feet on the floor.
- Keeping your abdominals braced, separate your hands to push your elbows towards the floor.
- Keep pushing backwards with your elbows to retract your shoulders and lift your torso away from the floor.
- Initially keep your bottom and feet on the floor, lifting only your torso.
- Hold for 3–5 seconds before returning to the start position.
- Repeat this 'lifting' technique 10–15 times.

Modifications

- To intensify this exercise, lift your bottom and torso so that just your elbows and feet are touching the floor.
- To intensify this exercise further, position your feet further away to increase the lever length.
- This can be progressed by extending your legs all the way to a straight-leg position and then even placing your feet on a BOSU.

Ex 7.23 Single-arm rows

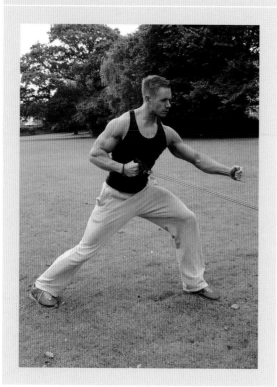

- As you pull, ensure you do not lean further back but maintain a fixed and braced position.
- As the grips near your ribcage, pause briefly before returning to the start position.
- Repeat 12–20 times before changing hands and repeating, holding the handles in your left hand.

Modifications

- Perform the pulling technique with alternate hands, but as the resistance is less, move further away from the fixed point to ensure suitable resistance.
- To add instability, perform this movement on one leg or even stand, sit or kneel on a BOSU, or sit on a stability ball.

Starting position and action

- Wrap a resistance tube around a tree trunk, post or similar secure anchor point, such as a door handle.
- Stand facing the anchor point with your feet shoulder-width apart, holding both handles of the resistance tube in your right hand with your palm facing inwards at chest height.
- Brace your abdominals and lean back with feet in a neutral or slightly split-stance, leaning back to take the strain.
- Pull back from your elbows and retract your shoulder blades, contracting your back and biceps muscles to pull the grips to your chest.

Ex 7.24 Prone stability ball pull-throughs

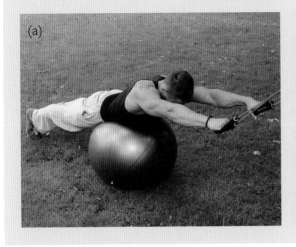

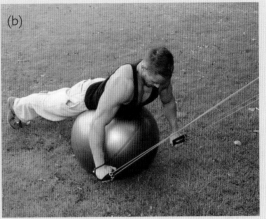

Starting position and action

- Secure a resistance tube around a tree, post, door handle or similar secure anchor point.
- Lie face down over a stability ball, holding the grips of the resistance tube in both hands with arms extended in front of you in line with your shoulders (Ex 7.24a).
- Maintaining abdominal tension, pull the handles down in an arc movement, keeping your elbows slightly locked to pull the grips underneath and behind you in an 'inverted pull-over' – essentially a 'pull-under' (Ex 7.24b).
- Keeping your arms slightly bent, return the grips back to the start position with your arms extended and in line with your shoulders.
- Ensure you keep your body position fixed throughout, without trying to lift the hips or adding any unnecessary force or momentum.

Modifications

- The angle of pull can be adjusted, as can the body position, and it is possible to perform this movement in a prone-incline position on the stability ball, pulling down, with the anchor point of the resistance tubes raised to a higher position.

EXERCISES FOR SHOULDERS

Ex 7.25 Single-arm curl and presses

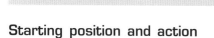

Starting position and action
- Stand in an upright position on a resistance tube, holding the grips in your right hand with the palm facing away from you and your arms by your side.
- Brace your abdominals and with your knees slightly bent, curl the grips towards you, bringing your hand to your shoulder.
- In this position, pause briefly and then extend your arm, pushing the grips upwards as you rotate your hand to face forwards, with your arm extended overhead.
- From this position, lower the grips slowly bringing your arm back to shoulder height and then lowering your hand to waist height.
- Repeat this curl and press movement 12–20 times before changing hands and repeating with your left hand.

Ex 7.26 Stability ball prone military presses

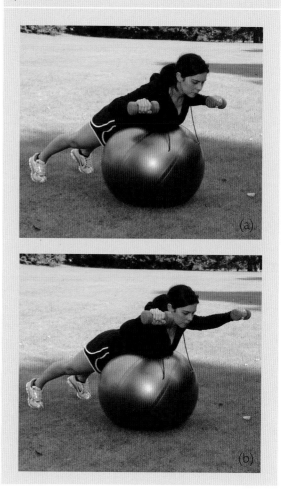

Starting position and action
- Kneel behind a stability ball and lie face down over the ball.
- Straighten your legs so that your abdominals and ribs are on the ball with feet acting as an anchor on the floor, hip-distance apart, keeping abdominals and glutes contracted.
- Holding of a pair of light dumbbells in each hand, extend your back and lift the dumb-

bells in line with your shoulders, keeping your abdominals braced throughout and your head in neutral alignment with your torso.

- Press the dumbbells over your head so that they travel 45–60 degrees to the floor.
- Hold very briefly when your arms are fully extended and then return the dumbbells back to shoulder height.
- Repeat 10–15 times before returning the dumbbells to the floor and resting.
- Do not lose correct form for increased resistance as you will find that fatigue can be achieved with resistance as low as 2–5kg.
- It is important to keep the back extended and abdominals braced, but do not hyperextend as this can aggravate your lower back.

Modification

- To intensify this exercise, position your feet closer together and perform the entire movement more slowly, rather than increasing the resistance.

Ex 7.27 Lateral raises

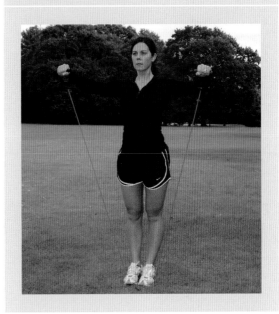

Starting position and action

- Hold a resistance tube by the grips in each hand, with your arms by your sides, and stand on the middle of the tube with both feet, keeping them together.
- Brace your abdominals and with your knees slightly bent lift your arms to the side, up to shoulder level, keeping your elbows slightly bent.
- Pause briefly in this raised position before slowly lowering your hands to your hips.
- Repeat 12–20 times.

Modifications

- To intensify this exercise, separate your feet to hip-distance apart.
- Cross the tube grips to opposite hands to increase the intensity.
- To reduce the intensity, stand on the tube with one leg only and bend your leg slightly.

Ex 7.28 Single-arm stability ball dumbbell presses

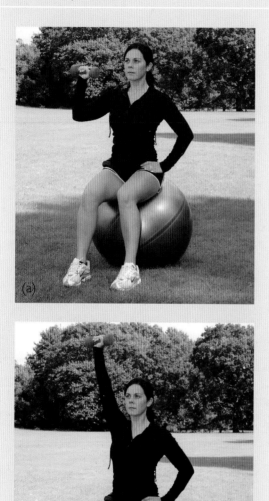

(a)

(b)

Starting position and action

- Begin holding a dumbbell at shoulder height while sitting on a stability ball with your feet shoulder-width apart and your abdominals braced.
- Maintain correct upright body alignment and press the dumbbell over your head, ensuring you do not lean or twist.
- Keep your left arm free and held loosely in front of your abdomen.
- Pause briefly in the overhead position before lowering back to your shoulder.
- Repeat shoulder press 12–15 times before changing hands and repeating on your left side.

Modifications

- While the unilateral element to this exercise makes this challenging enough for your core, to increase the stabilisation requirement, try raising one foot off the floor, as this really challenges your core muscles and stabilisation.
- To reduce the intensity, place your feet wider than shoulder-width apart to assist your balance and reduce the stabilisation required.

EXERCISES FOR LEGS

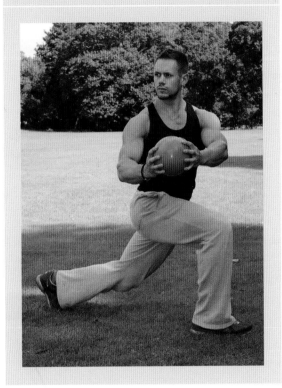

Ex 7.29 Forward lunges with trunk rotation

Starting position and action

- Begin standing upright with your arms outstretched at chest height holding a medicine ball.
- Step forwards with your right leg into a lunge position so that as your foot strikes the floor you bend both knees and lower down until your front (right) thigh is almost parallel to the floor.
- Your rear knee should bend but not touch the floor.

- As you lower, rotate your torso 90 degrees to your right side, twisting at the waist.
- Maintain correct posture throughout, keeping your abdominals braced throughout the movement, and do not hold your breath at any point.
- Slowly rotate back to the start position, and contract your glutes, hamstrings and quad muscles of your right leg and buttocks, to lift you back to a standing position.
- In a continuous action, take a step forward with your left leg and as your left foot touches the floor, bend your knees and lower towards the floor. Rotate to your left side until your left thigh is almost parallel to the floor and your torso is fully rotated with arms outstretched, holding the medicine ball and pointing to the left.
- Continue to lunge forwards with alternate legs and rotating to alternate sides. Keep your arms outstretched, holding the ball parallel to the floor.
- Keep your torso upright throughout the movement and maintain abdominal tension throughout.
- Repeat lunge action and rotation 10–20 times.

Ex 7.30 Side lunges with medicine ball pick-ups*

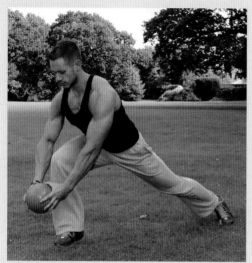

* Image shows modification

Starting position and action

- Stand with feet shoulder-width apart holding a medicine ball with both hands.
- Keeping your abdominals braced, initially take a sideways lunge out to your right side into a lateral lunge position.
- Bend your right knee to 'sit' further into the lunge position and then, reaching down with your arms, place the medicine ball on the floor.
- Maintaining abdominal bracing, push off your right leg, contracting your quads, hamstrings and gluteal muscles to return back to the start position.
- Then step out again into a sideways lunge with your right leg, to return to the last position so that you can reach the medicine ball.
- 'Sit' down into the lunge position so that you can pick up the medicine ball, and, bracing your abdominals, push back, contracting your quads, hamstrings and gluteal muscles to return to the start position.
- Repeat this place-and-retrieve movement 10–15 times before changing to your left, repeating again 10–15 times.
- This exercise can also be performed with dumbells.

Modification 1: Multi-direction lunges with medicine ball pick-ups

- Lunge out at varying angles, not just laterally, but forwards, diagonally and backwards.
- Ideally, consider a clock face, imagining 12 o'clock being straight in front of you and 6 o'clock being directly behind you.
- Aim to put down and collect the medicine ball working around a clock face in any order, e.g. 6 o'clock, 2 o'clock, 8 o'clock, 3 o'clock, etc.

Modification 2: Multi-direction lunges with dumbell curl and press

- As you lower into the lunge position, curl the dumbbell towards your shoulder and then in the lowest part of the lunge, maintain the position and press the dumbbell overhead.
- Pause briefly at the top position and then lower the dumbbell back to the shoulder and as you push back to the upright position, lower the dumbbell back to the hips.
- Repeat 6–10 times before changing the dumbbell to the opposite hand and leading with the opposite leg.

Ex 7.31 Lunge and pulls

Modification

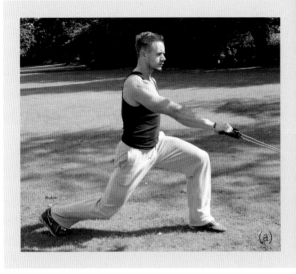

(a)

Starting position and action

- Secure a resistance tube around a post or similar so that you are holding a single handle in your right hand.
- Step/lunge forward with your left leg approximately a stride length in front of you.
- As your left leg touches the floor, bend your left knee and drop into a forward lunge position.
- Ensure as you do this that your abdominals are fully braced and that you are in an upright posture.
- As you lower towards the floor, decelerate the movement, ensuring you do not lean forwards.
- When you are in the full lunge position, drive back with your left leg by contracting through your glutes and thigh muscles to push you back with sufficient force to the start position.
- As you reach the start position, pull the resistance tube handle, using your back and arm muscles to draw the handle to your ribs.

- Pause briefly before repeating this complete movement and lunging forwards again on to your left leg.
- Repeat 10–15 times before changing hands and repeating, this time lunging forwards with your right leg.

Modifications

- Initially this exercise should be done slowly and under control, but it can be performed dynamically and at pace.
- Care should be taken to really brace your abdominals, to avoid any unnecessary forward lean during the lunge stage.
- As you propel yourself back to the start position, a nice variation is to step back with your lunging leg as you pull the handle to your ribs. This acts as a breaking and stabilising action and allows you to generate a smooth cadence of dynamic lunging and rowing with slight body rotation.

Ex 7.32 Step-ups to balance with overhead press

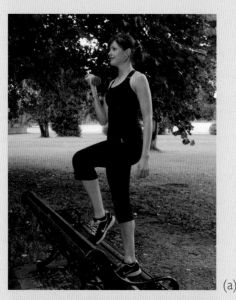

(a)

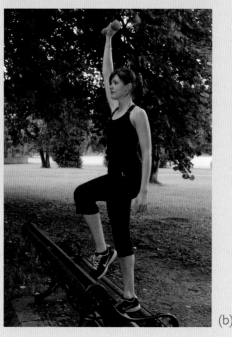

(b)

Starting position and action

- Stand behind a bench or a raised wall holding a dumbbell in your right hand with your arms by your sides.
- Brace your abdominals and step up on to the bench, leading with your right leg.
- As your left leg draws near the bench, flex your left knee at the hip and lift your left thigh until it is almost horizontal.
- Simultaneously curl the dumbbell in your right hand towards your right shoulder and then press it overhead.
- Pause briefly at the 'upper' position with your left leg raised and hold your balance, before lowering the dumbbell back to shoulder height and then lower to your hips.
- As the dumbbell returns, flex your right leg and step back with your left leg to lower yourself back to the floor and step back down with your right leg.
- Repeat 10–12 times, leading with your right leg before transferring the dumbbell to your left hand and repeating the movement, this time leading with the left leg.
- It is important not to use a weight that is too heavy until you have mastered the technique.

Modification

- It is possible to vary which hand you hold the dumbbell in in relation to your lead leg, i.e. step up with your right leg holding the dumbbell in your right hand, or hold the dumbbell in the opposite hand to your lead leg. This will affect both your co-ordination and balance.

Ex 7.33 Overhead dumbbell squats with rotation

(a)

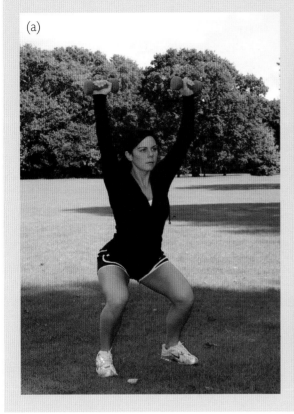

(b)

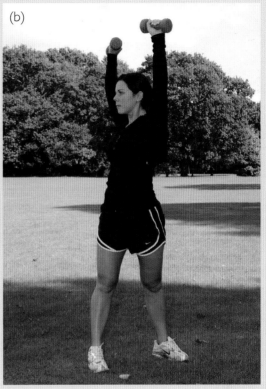

Starting position and action

- Begin in a neutral stance, feet parallel, holding a pair of dumbbells overhead.
- Maintain correct upright posture and brace your abdominals.
- Squat down by bending your knees to sit down into a squat position with dumbbells raised above your head.
- Pause briefly at the lowest point, when your thighs are almost parallel to the floor, before extending through your knees and hips back to standing position.

- As you return to the standing position, rotate 90 degrees to your right side.
- Then squat down again, facing forwards when you reach the full squat position before pushing back up to a standing position, this time by rotating 90 degrees to your left.
- Repeat alternate squats and rotations 12–20 times before lowering dumbbells to the floor.

Ex 7.34 Hip thrusts

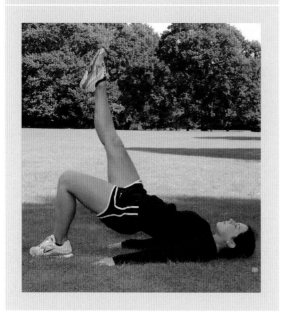

Ex 7.35 Power hops

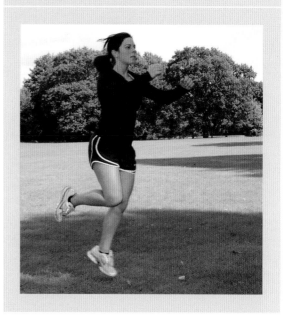

Starting position and action

- Lie on your back with your knees bent and lift your right leg into the air above your hips.
- Brace your abdominals and squeezing your glutes and the hamstrings of your left leg, push your hips upwards without twisting.
- At the upper position, pause briefly before lowering back towards to the floor slowly. Just before your buttocks touch the floor, push upwards by activating your glutes and hamstrings to repeat the lift.
- Repeat 10–15 times with your right leg raised and then change position and repeat, this time with your left leg raised.
- This is an excellent exercise for glute strength and hip stability.

Starting position and action

- Position marker cones 10–20m apart and stand on your left leg, keeping it slightly bent, ready to hop.
- Bend your leg and then push off to hop forwards towards the marker cone.
- Use your arms to assist your jump and keeping your torso upright, push off your left leg repeatedly to cover the distance.
- On reaching the marker cone, walk back to the start position and repeat the drill on your right leg.
- Repeat this drill 3–5 times for each leg, aiming to hop with fewer hops over the distance for each attempt. This increases the intensity and power requirement of the drill and is an excellent drill for dynamic power in your legs.
- If you do not have marker cones, just use a sweatshirt or similar.

EXERCISES FOR ARMS

Ex 7.36 Biceps curls

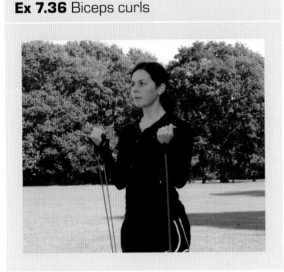

Ex 7.37 Kneeling triceps extension

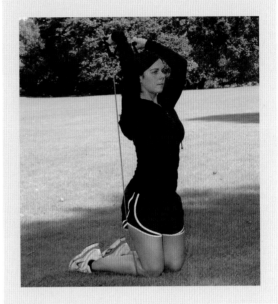

Starting position and action

- Stand on a resistance tube with both feet, holding a handle in each hand.
- With palms facing away from you, while maintaining abdominal tension and your knees slightly bent, curl the tube handles towards your chest.
- Pause briefly in the top position before slowly lowering the grips back to the start position.
- Repeat biceps curls 15–20 times.

Modifications

- To reduce the intensity, stand on the resistance tube with one leg or bend your legs slightly.
- To increase the resistance either use two tubes, to double the intensity or stand in a wider stance to increase the resistance stretch on the tube.

Starting position and action

- Kneel on the resistance tube, holding a handle in each hand, with your elbows pointing upwards and hands by your shoulders, with palms up.
- Maintain correct body alignment and brace your abdominals as you extend both arms overhead
- Pause briefly at full extension with arms overhead, before lowering the handles back to shoulder height.
- Repeat triceps extensions overhead for 15–20 repetitions, ensuring your hips are stabilised and your spine is in neutral.

EXAMPLE GARDEN WORKOUTS

While Part 3 incorporates numerous environments and possible exercise choices to suit each of them, bodyweight exercise is not dependent upon one specific environment only. As such, exercises from the garden, beach, park, urban, bootcamp or buggy workout could be incorporated into other workouts. In addition, each activity is largely dependent on the space and available equipment and fitness of the individual. Tables 7.1 and 7.2 show examples of possible

Table 7.1	Cardio and resistance mixed circuit			
Ex no.	Page	Exercise	Repetitions	Option I circuit Complete all exercises in order
Warm-up	14	Warm-up variations (see chapter 3)		
7.1	58	Jumping jacks	30–45 sec	1/16
7.16	67	Push-ups on your knees	15–20	2/17
7.24	73	Prone stability ball pull-through	15–20	3/18
7.3	59	Kangaroos	30–45 sec	4/19
7.28	76	Single-arm stability ball dumbbell shoulder press	15–20	5/20
7.31	79	Lunge and pull	15–20	6/21
7.4	59	Squat thrusts	30–45 sec	7/22
7.22	71	Supine shoulder retractions	15–20	8/23
7.32	80	Step-up to balance with overhead press	15–20	9/24
7.35	82	Power hops	30–45 sec	10/25
7.36	83	Biceps curls	15–25	11/26
7.37	83	Alternate triceps press	15–25	12/27
7.2	58	Air jacks	30–45 sec	13/28
7.20	70	Stability ball cobra	10–15	14/29
7.8	62	Dynamic planks	30–45 sec	15/30
	237–40	Cool-down and stretch		

Table 7.2		Peripheral heart action circuit		
Ex no.	**Page**	**Exercise**	**Repetitions**	**Option 1 circuit (3 circuits)** Complete all exercises in order
Warm-up	14–27	Warm-up variations (see chapter 3)		
7.11	64	Stability ball roll-outs	10–15	1/13/25
7.29	77	Forward lunge with trunk rotation	15–20	2/14/26
7.17	68	Push-ups with rotation	15–20	3/15/27
7.30	78	Side lunges with medicine ball pick-up	15–20	4/16/28
7.23	72	Single-arm row	15–20	5/17/29
7.31	79	Lunge and pull	15–20	6/18/30
7.26	74	Stability ball prone military press	15–20	7/19/31
7.32	130	Step-up with overhead press	15–20	8/20/32
7.34	82	Hip thrusts	15–20	9/21/33
7.33	81	Overhead dumbbell squat with rotation	15–20	10/22/34
7.14	66	Super-slow bicycles	15–25	11/23/35
7.35	82	Power hops	15–25	12/24/36
	237–40	Cool-down and stretch		

exercise choices that might be applicable within a garden workout, but feel free to incorporate exercises from the other sections as required. Within the Appendices (*see* p. 233) you will find a full list of suitable post-workout stretches, together with some examples of self-myofasicial release (SMR) stretches, if you have specific tightness in certain muscles.

Table 7.3 gives different options for circuit workouts incorporating a basic circuit (Option 1) whereby you simply follow the exercises in order to the bottom (A14) before repeating at the top for the second circuits (A15). Option 2 applies a super-set and tri-set workout whereby you would complete all the A exercises in order before moving on to the next cardio exercise and then working through all the B exercises in order. To clarify, this would mean completing: abdominal bridge, stability ball back extension, back to abdominal bridge and then stability ball back extension before completing the cardio exercise – jumping jacks.

Option 3 is a giant-set workout in which you complete three sets of all the A exercises: abdominal bridge, back extension, jumping jacks, single-arm dumbbell press and single-arm row before beginning again with abdominal bridge. This principle applies all the way through completing all the A exercises three times, then all the B exercises three times, etc.

Table 7.3		Agonist/antagonist (opposing muscle groups) and cardio interval workout			
Ex no.	Page	Exercise 15–25 repetitions unless otherwise stated	Option 1 circuit Complete exercises in order	Option 2 super-sets Perform exercises alternately (A/B/C/D/E)	Option 3 giant sets/ mini circuit Perform exercises 2–3 times in blocks (A/B/C)
Warm-up	14–27	Warm-up variations (see chapter 3)			
7.5	60	Abdominal bridges (planks) (hold 30 sec)	A1/A15	A1/A3	A1/A6/A11
7.21	71	Stability ball back extension	A2/A16	A2/A4	A2/A7/A12
7.1	58	Jumping jacks (30 sec to 1 min)	A3/A17	Jumping Jacks	A3/A8/A13
7.28	76	Single-arm stability ball dumbbell press	A4/A18	B1/ B3/B5	A4/A9/A14
7.23	72	Single-arm row	A5/A19	B2/B4/B6	A5/A10/A15
7.2	58	Air jacks (30 sec to 1 min)	A6/A20	Air jacks	B1/B7
7.25	74	Single-arm curl and press	A7/A21	C1/C3/C5	B2/B8
7.29	77	Forward lunge with trunk rotation	A8/A22	C2/C4/C6	B3/B9
7.35	82	Power hops (1 min)	A9/A23	Power hops	B4/B10
7.36	83	Biceps curls	A10/A24	D1/D3/D5	B5/B11
9.3	138	Bench dips	A11/A25	D2/D4/D6	B6/B12
7.4	59	Squat thrusts (30 sec to 1 min)	A12/A26	Squat thrusts	C1/C4/C7
7.6	60	Abdominal curls on stability ball	A13/A27	E1/E3	C2/C5/C8
7.3	59	Kangaroos	A14/A28	E2/E4	C3/C6/C9
	237–40	Cool-down and stretch			

BEACH WORKOUT

8

If you have the opportunity of using a beach to train on – whether you are on holiday or you live near the coast, there are many exercises drills that you can create to suit your environment. A beach workout can be just a bit of fun with your kids or a hardcore total-body workout, it's up to you.

Firstly, check out what's available – use your imagination and your surroundings for anything that you can jump over, lift, push against or even race with. Use your bodyweight for many of the resistance exercises and if you can bring along a towel or resistance tube, all the better. If your overall goal is to tone up and improve your fitness, anything that makes you breathless and is continuous will not only train your aerobic system but will burn calories and ultimately help burn fat as well. But remember: even though working out on a beach might look appealing, be aware of the terrain – you might be surprised how challenging running up a sand dune or pebble beach is in comparison to a road or grassy hill, and if you are exercising on sandy stretches of beach, always be aware of the changing tides.

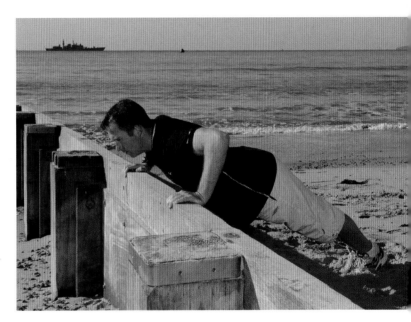

Remember to warm up by taking a brisk walk or jog along the beach and include some of the mobilisation and dynamic stretches suggested in chapter 3. This chapter includes predominantly bodyweight and some partner-resistance exercises to keep the equipment minimal. You could include some of the footwork drills from chapter 4 by carving a speed ladder in the sand, or use any exercises shown in previous or subsequent chapters to complement your overall workout.

CARDIO AND AGILITY DRILLS

Ex 8.1 Breakwater hurdles

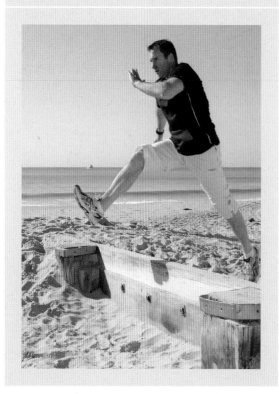

Ex 8.2 Breakwater up-and-overs

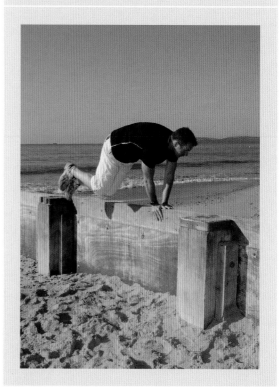

Starting position and action

- Look for a breakwater of moderate height that has an equal drop on either side.
- Stand 5–10m away from the breakwater and take a run-up in preparation to jump over it in a hurdling action.
- Hurdle or jump over the breakwater, turning around after each jump and repeating from the other direction for 10–15 hurdles.

Starting position and action

- Stand on one side of a wooden breakwater, holding the top with both hands.
- With your feet together and your knees slightly bent, brace your abdominals and push off your legs to propel your legs and hips into the air, while holding on to the breakwater, to 'jump' from one side of it to the other.
- As you land on the other side, cushion your landing by bending your knees before pushing back up with your legs to 'jump' over to the other side of the breakwater.
- Repeat these jumps over the breakwater for 30–45 seconds.

Ex 8.3 Beach sprints

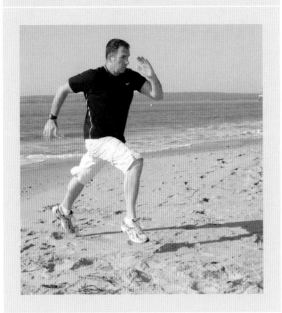

Ex 8.4 Surf shuttles

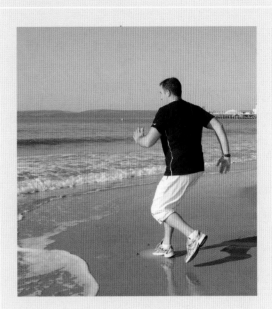

Starting position and action

- Depending upon your beach terrain – pebbles or sand – these sprints are excellent interval-training options.
- Start at the bottom of a sand dune or at the lowest point on a pebble beach.
- With a rapid and dynamic arm action and fast leg movement, sprint up the sand dune or up the pebbles to the top, keeping your arms bent at 90 degrees and driving forwards, lifting your knees high in a fast sprinting action.
- At the top of the beach or sand dune, turn around and walk or jog back down to the lowest point on the beach before sprinting up to the top of the beach again.
- Repeat sprint 5–10 times. The effect of the loose pebbles or sand makes the sprinting action much harder, as your footing is compromised.

Starting position and action

- This is an 'opportunistic interval' and works really well with children or working against a partner for fun.
- You have to 'create' the interval based on the tide and the waves on the shore, in a similar fashion to that depicted in the 'Monkees Theme' video, by The Monkees pop group from the 1960s.
- Start by setting a point to start from, facing the sea and then sprinting/accelerating towards the waves as they break on the shore.
- Before the wave reaches you (as you run towards it), rapidly change direction to run away from the wave before you get your feet wet.
- Repeat these 'surf shuttles' 10–20 times before resting.

Ex 8.5 Burpees

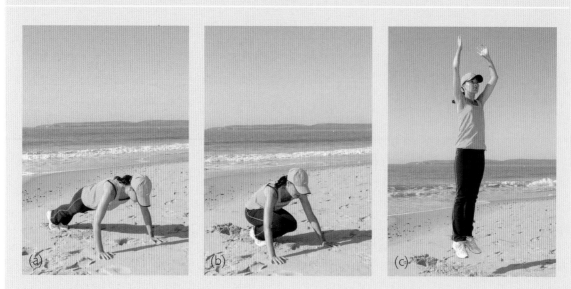

Starting position and action

- Begin standing upright with your feet hip-distance apart and arms by your sides.
- Squat down to place your hands on the floor, shoulder-width apart and slightly in front of your feet.
- Keeping your abdominals braced, take your weight on to your arms and drive both feet back into an extended position, to land with both feet at the same time ensuring you are not dropping your hips but keeping your pelvis and back stabilised (8.5a).
- From the extended position, lean into your arms to take more of your bodyweight again as you push off your toes and drive your knees in towards your chest (8.5b).
- Then push yourself back on to your feet as you and stand up, in the start position.
- Repeat this 'squat thrust and stand up' movement 20–50 times.

Modifications

- When in the prone extended position, with arms shoulder-width apart, keep your abdominals braced and to perform a push-up, by bending your arms.
- As your chest nears the floor, extend your arms to return back to the prone position before pushing off your toes and drawing your knees in, as before. Push yourself back on to your feet and stand up to the start position.
- Repeat burpee movement with a push-up for 20–30 repetitions or for a timed period of 45 seconds to 1 minute.
- An alternative is to add a jump as you stand up after each burpee (8.5c).

Ex 8.6 Falling starts

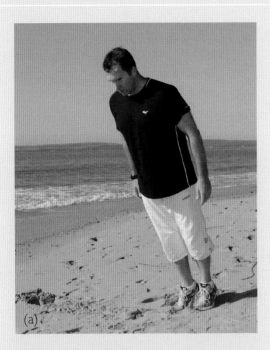

(a)

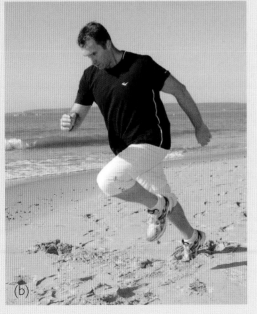

(b)

Starting position and action

- Begin standing upright with your arms by your sides in a relaxed posture.
- Lift up on to your toes and lean forwards, keeping your torso and legs in alignment.
- Allow yourself to 'fall forwards' until the very last moment when you 'react' by driving upwards with your arms and pushing off your legs in a sprinting action to accelerate forwards over 20–30m.
- After completing the desired distance, decelerate comfortably down to a walking speed and then either jog or walk back to the start position and repeat 5–8 times.
- The emphasis in this drill is to lean beyond the point of 'no return' and accelerate at the last moment safely into a sprint action.

EXERCISES FOR THE CORE

Ex 8.7 Resistance tube woodchops

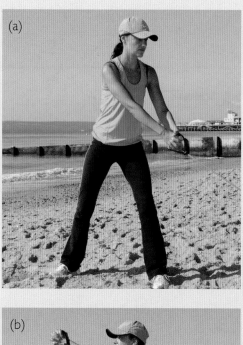
(a)

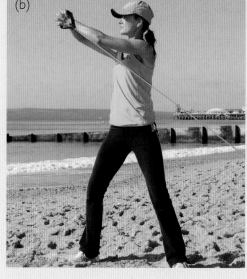
(b)

Starting position and action

- Wrap a resistance tube around a breakwater or railing and take hold of both grips, holding with your hands clasped together.
- Stand sideways to the 'anchor point' and bend your legs, bracing your abdominals.
- Twist from your waist in a smooth action, away from the anchor point to stretch the resistance tube, keeping your arms in a fixed position while holding the handles.
- Do not 'over rotate' in this movement or use a resistance that compromises your technique.
- Repeat 10–15 times before turning to face the opposite direction and rotating again away from the anchor point to work your opposite side.

Modifications

- This exercise can be performed from a kneeling position to minimise hip and leg involvement.
- For a sports-specific application, try kneeling on one leg with your other foot on the floor, as in a canoeing stance.
- It is good to vary the anchor point so as to work the core muscles in different directions. Also try changing the start and finish point of the movement, the angle and the direction of pull.
- You can vary the resistance by holding just one handle of the resistance tube, with the other end secured, or even by using two resistance tubes for extra resistance.
- It is important to maintain tension in the tube and never allow any slack by standing too close to the anchor point.
-

Ex 8.8 Slow eccentric abdominal curls

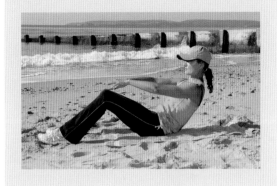

Ex 8.9 Spiderman walk

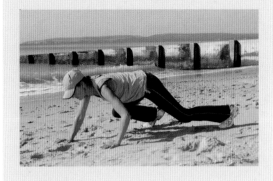

Starting position and action

- Lie on the ground with your knees bent over your hips, your hands holding the backs of your thighs and your feet in the air.
- Rock yourself forward, to assist you in the sit-up technique and bring your feet on to the ground in a near-seated position.
- Reach forwards with your arms so that your hands are over your knees with arms straight.
- To maintain this position, contract your abdominals, and then slowly roll down through the spine over 10–20 seconds to lower yourself down to the ground until your shoulders return to the floor.
- Then raise your legs as before and repeat 5–10 times, keeping the lowering movement slow.

Modifications

- To increase the difficulty and the resistance, place your arms across your chest, or for a greater challenge, keep your hands behind your head.

Starting position and action

- Position yourself on 'all fours' with your weight evenly spread between your feet and your hands.
- Brace your abdominals and keep your torso as rigid as possible.
- Keep your feet and knees 'turned out' slightly to minimise hip-flexor involvement and spinal movement.
- Crawl forwards, taking small steps with your hands and feet yet with minimal movement through your hips and pelvis.
- Aim to cover a distance of 10–20m, before resting briefly and repeating.

Ex 8.10 Horizontal balance

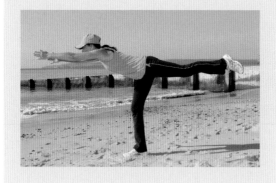

Ex 8.11 Abdominal scissor curls

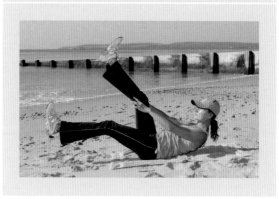

Starting position and action

- Bend your supporting right leg slightly and begin to slowly lean forwards, keeping your abdominals braced.
- As you continue to flex at your hip by leaning forwards, lift your left leg, trying to keep this leg in line with your torso.
- Lift your arms so that your arms, torso and left leg are all in line and aim to lean forwards until you reach a horizontal position.
- Hold this position for 10–15 seconds before slowly returning to the start position.
- Repeat 5–8 times before changing your balance to your left leg and then repeating the entire movement, this time balancing on your left leg and raising your right leg as you lean.

Starting position and action

- Lie on your back with both legs raised in the air at about 70–80 degrees, your shoulders and upper back should be off the ground as you reach your arms towards your toes.
- Hold this position as you slowly lower your right leg so that your heel almost touches the ground, then raise your right leg towards your hands while simultaneously lowering your left leg down to almost touch the ground in a scissor action.
- Maintain abdominal tension throughout this movement and repeat this scissor action, alternating legs for 20–30 repetitions.

Modifications

- This drill can be performed in a partial curl-up position, alternately you can maintain a braced neutral spine position with your shoulders on the ground, but don't allow the movement of your legs to compromise this abdominal tension and neutral spine.

Ex 8.12 Lateral bridging*

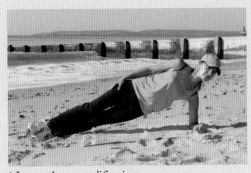

*Image shows modification

Ex 8.13 Two-point prone bridges

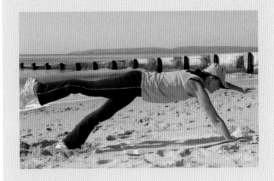

Starting position and action

- Lie on your left side with knees bent, heels behind you, and rest on your left elbow and forearm – your elbow should be directly underneath the shoulder.
- Brace your abdominals and lift your hips up keeping your knees, hips and torso in line.
- Maintain the tension through the abdominals and hold for 10–20 seconds.
- Do not allow the shoulder to lose tension as this can cause pain in the neck area.
- Lower your hips to the floor for a very brief recovery and repeat, aiming for 10–15 repetitions before lying on your left side and repeating the exercise.

Modifications

- To intensify this exercise, extend your legs and lift, keeping your torso and legs in line and rigid, your weight being supported through your elbow, forearm and the side of your foot.
- Maintain abdominal tension throughout and do not allow your body to sag.

Starting position and action

- Begin initially in a push-up position but with hands placed shoulder-width apart and your arms straight.
- Keeping your abdominals braced, simultaneously lift both your left arm and right leg off the floor.
- Aim to keep the knee of the raised leg level with the hips, shoulders and raised arm, holding this position for 5–10 seconds before lowering back to the start position.
- Repeat the exercise with your opposite arm and leg for 8–12 complete repetitions with each limb.

Modifications

- This two-point bridge can be modified by performing a press-up, but as you push yourself away from the floor, lift your leg and opposite arm to considerably intensify this exercise.

Ex 8.14 Impossible bridges

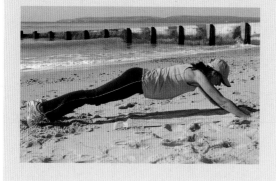

Starting position and action
- This is an advanced position and very challenging to your core and shoulder muscles.
- Begin lying face down on the floor with your arms outstretched in front of you with palms down and your toes on the floor.
- Bracing your abdominals, push down hard with your arms and lift your hips (15–40cm) off the floor.
- You might need to adjust your footing slightly by walking your toes in to reduce the intensity.
- This is a very intense exercise, so hold the position for 2–5 seconds before lowering back to the start.
- Repeat 5–10 times.

Ex 8.15 Reverse curls

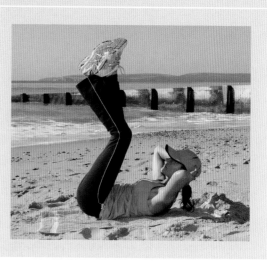

Starting position and action
- Lie down on a towel on the sand face up, with your knees flexed and over your hips and your ankles crossed.
- Either place your arms by your sides, with palms up or place your hands behind your head.
- Slowly tilt your pelvis, lifting your hips towards the ceiling in a controlled manner so that your knees move towards your chest.
- Pause briefly at the top phase before slowly lowering the hips back to the floor.
- Try not to swing your knees in this movement. Aim for a controlled abdominal contraction and slow movement throughout.
- Repeat 15–30 times.

Ex 8.16 Oblique crunches

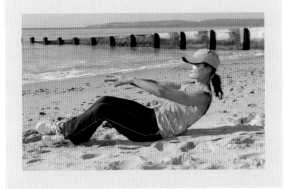

Starting position and action

- Lie down on a towel with your knees bent and feet together on the floor.
- Cross your left leg over your right ankle and lower both knees to the left towards the floor at an angle of between 30 and 45 degrees to the ground.
- Lift your head slightly so that you can see that your chin, right hip and ankles are in line.
- With both hands reaching forwards over your right hip, curl upwards, reaching towards your ankles and pausing briefly at the top position before lowering back to the ground.
- Repeat 15–20 times before repeating on the other side, this time the right leg crosses over the left ankle and the knees drop down towards your right.

Ex 8.17 Breakwater balance drills

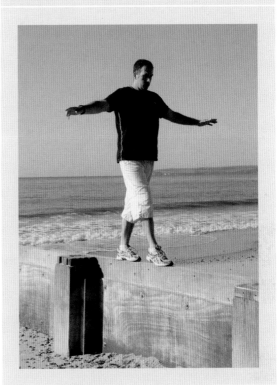

Starting position and action

- Choose a low breakwater that you will not hurt yourself from should you fall.
- Carefully step up on to the breakwater and begin to slowly walk along the wooden edge, maintaining your balance.
- To add difficulty, try turning 180 degrees while balancing and then walk back.
- Continue this walking balance for between 30 seconds and 1 minute.

EXERCISES FOR THE CHEST

Ex 8.18 Breakwater push-ups

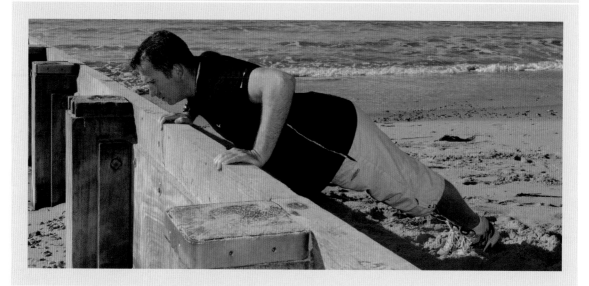

Starting position and action

- Find a suitable breakwater or wall to lean on so that your bodyweight is supported through your arms, with your legs outstretched behind you.
- Position your hands slightly wider than shoulder-width apart, keeping your torso stabilised and legs straight, with your spine in neutral alignment.
- Bracing your abdominals, lower your torso down towards the breakwater or low wall by bending your arms until your chest almost reaches the breakwater.
- Pause briefly at the lowest point and then extend your arms to return back to the start position.
- Repeat these breakwater push-ups 10–20 times before resting.

Modifications

- Depending upon the height of the breakwater, it might be possible to kneel on the sand to make the exercise easier. However, kneeling on pebbles might be too uncomfortable.
- Alternatively, to increase the intensity, try and find a lower breakwater so that more of your bodyweight is being supported through your arms.
- Depending upon the height of the breakwater and your own strength, you might want to try an inverted push-up, whereby your feet on the breakwater while your hands are on the sand/ pebbles. This is a much harder version and correct form should be maintained throughout.

Ex 8.19 Kneeling partner-resisted chest presses

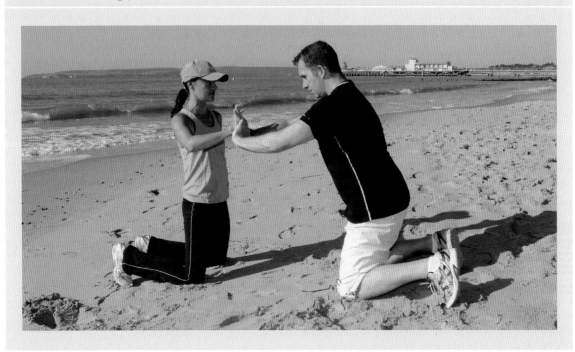

Starting position and action

- Working with a partner, kneel down on the ground in an upright position, keeping your spine in neutral alignment with your abdominals braced. Your partner should stand or kneel in front of you.
- Raise your right hand to your chest with your right elbow behind you and your palms facing your partner.
- Your partner places their hand or hands against your palm with their arms slightly bent in preparation for you to push against them.
- With your abdominals fully braced and keeping your torso still, push against your partner's hand as if performing a single-arm chest press.
- When you reach extension of the arm, your partner applies more pressure and you control this extra force by returning your arm, eccentrically working your chest, shoulder and triceps muscles.
- Repeat this single-arm chest press 10–15 times, maintaining correct abdominal pressure throughout and ensuring trunk and torso stability before changing arms and repeating.

Modifications

- It is important to maintain slow controlled movement for all partner resistance exercises. Avoid leaning into the movement and using your bodyweight as this is about core stabilisation and functional strength.
- If you do not have a partner, use a resistance tube, secured around a post or railing. Hold both grips in one hand.

Ex 8.20 Gecko crawl with push-ups

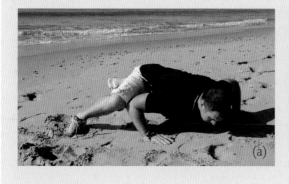
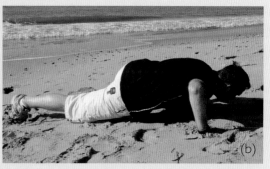

(a)   (b)

Starting position and action

- This is a very advanced push-up drill and requires both co-ordination and upper-body and torso strength.
- Begin in a push-up position with your arms extended and shoulder-width apart, with your feet together and abdominals braced.
- Still in the prone position, lift your right leg and, bending at the knee, bring your right foot up almost level with your left knee so that your right knee nears your right elbow.
- Simultaneously lift your left arm to place it about 10–20cm forwards, causing your hands to be in a split position and your torso flexed laterally to your right side.
- In this position, with feet and hands staggered, perform a push-up, lowering your chest to the floor.
- Push back up to an extended arm position and then lift your right arm and left leg together, placing your right hand about 10–20cm in front of your left.
- At the same time, bring your left foot up and place in front of your right foot so that your left knee is almost touching your left elbow with your torso laterally flexed to your left.
- In this position perform another push-up, keeping your abdominals braced throughout.
- Repeat these walking push-ups over a distance of 10m, before resting.
- The action and strange body movements causing you to perform push-ups in a flexed body position are 'lizard-like', hence the name.

Ex 8.21 Staggered push-ups

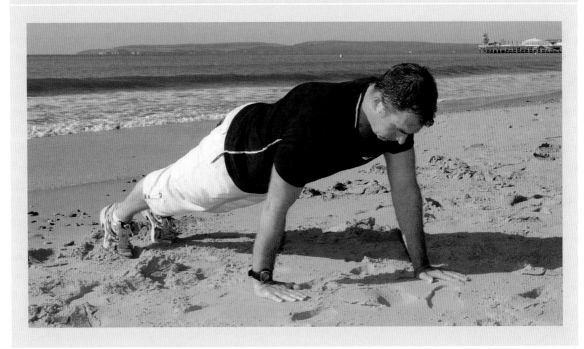

Starting position and action

- An easier push-up variation than the gecko crawl is to simply perform the push-up with a straight body but with the hands shoulder-width apart, and one hand in front of the other.
- Perform a push-up as normal and on completion reverse your hand position and repeat the push-up technique, repeating 15–25 times.

EXERCISES FOR THE BACK

Ex 8.22 Railing pull-ups

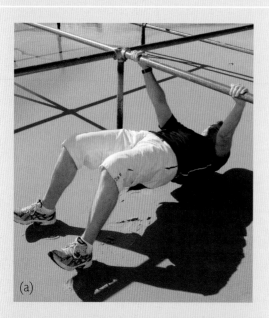

(a)

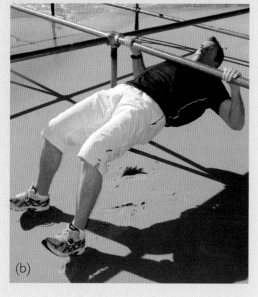

(b)

Starting position and action

- The pull-up is one the best upper body exercises, yet to perform a normal pull-up is often beyond the reach of many people.
- Find a railing suitable to hold on to with both hands and hang down with your arms extended, with your knees slightly bent and feet on the floor while you look up at the railing.
- Brace your abdominals and pull yourself upwards, bringing your chest towards the railing, pausing briefly at the top position with your shoulder blades retracted and arms flexed, before lowering back down to the start position.
- Repeat these hanging modified pull-ups 10–15 times.

Modifications

- To intensify the exercise, straighten your legs further to increase the lever length or even elevate your feet by placing them on a ball or low post or similar.

Ex 8.23 Back hyper-extension

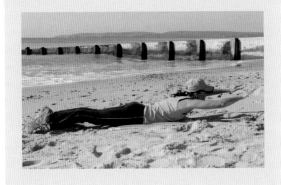

Starting position and action

- Lie face down on a towel on the sand with your arms outstretched above your head.
- Keep your legs slightly separated to assist stability.
- Extend through your back to lift your chest off the floor, keeping your head in neutral alignment, looking down.
- Rise up to lift your chest off the floor a few inches, pausing briefly in this raised position before lowering to the floor.
- Remember to tense your abdominals before initiating any movement and keep braced throughout. Avoid trying to lift too far and over-arching the back.
- Be careful not to twist the spine.
- Repeat 10–15 times, keeping the movement slow and controlled.

Modification

- You can reduce the intensity by bringing your hands next to your ears or having them by your sides to reduce the lever length.

Ex 8.24 Partner rows

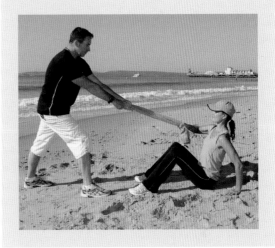

Starting position and action

- Sit down with your knees slightly bent and lean back, holding on to a towel in your right hand with your arm outstretched.
- Your partner should stand in a braced position holding the other end of the towel in front of you, making sure the towel is taut.
- Brace your abdominals and, gripping on to the towel, try and pull it towards you by pulling your right elbow back and behind you, keeping your thumb upwards.
- Retract your shoulders and pull the towel to approximately level with your ribs.
- Pause briefly and allow your partner to provide a little more resistance as you return to the start position.
- Repeat using your right arm for 12–15 repetitions and then change to your left side.
- It is important to keep the pulling action slow and controlled and talk to your partner to encourage the correct amount of resistance or pulling.

EXERCISES FOR SHOULDERS

Ex 8.25 Upright rows

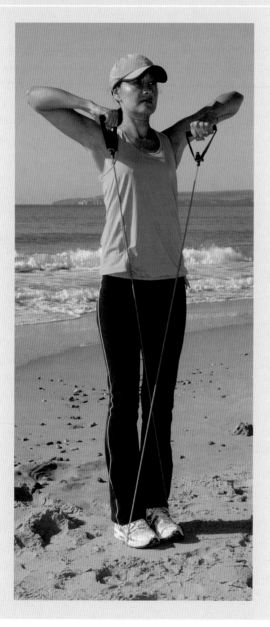

Starting position and action

- Stand on the resistance tube with your feet together, holding a handle in each hand, palms facing towards you and with the tube crossed in front of your legs.
- Keeping your abdominals braced and your knees slightly bent, lift the handles, leading with your elbows until your hands are approximately shoulder height, with your elbows pointing upwards by your ears.
- Pause briefly in this top position and then lower your hands slowly back to the start position.
- Repeat rows 12–20 times.

Modifications

- To intensify this exercise, stand on the tube with your feet hip-distance apart.
- If you needed to reduce the intensity, stand on the tube with one leg, and to reduce intensity further, bend this leg slightly to reduce the stretch in the tube.

Ex 8.26 Partner-resisted lateral raises

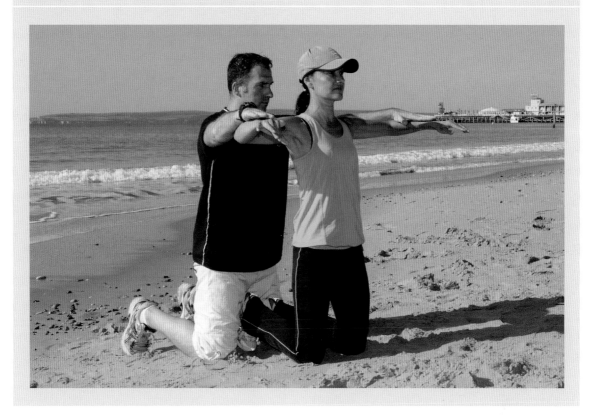

Starting position and action

- Have your partner kneel or stand behind you with their hands on your elbows and/or forearms as you kneel down on the sand.
- Keeping your abdominals braced with your knees apart, raise your arms to the side slowly to almost shoulder height, keeping your elbows slightly bent.
- Your partner should be pressing your elbows against the direction of movement, initially in towards your torso and as you lift your arms, downwards to provide suitable resistance.
- Pause briefly in this top position and then allow your partner to apply greater resistance as you

lower eccentrically, against the increased resistance of your partner, back to the start position.
- Repeat 10–15 times.

Modifications

- Depending upon your strength and that of your partner, they might need to apply the resistance as low down as your wrists if you are much stronger, as this increased lever length will make it easier for them.
- If this is the case it might be easier for them to stand or kneel in front of you, as with your arms slightly flexed, it might become awkward to apply resistance from behind.

EXERCISES FOR LEGS

Ex 8.27 Squat walks

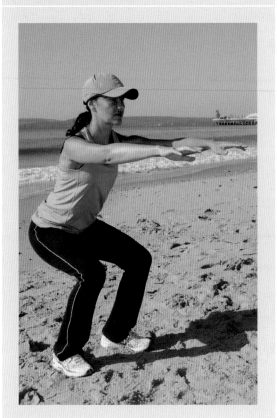

do so. Keep your abdominals braced and spine in neutral.

- Then extend your legs and hips to return back to a standing position.
- From this new standing position, take a pace forwards with both legs before squatting down as before until both thighs are parallel to the ground.
- Extend your legs and hips to return to a standing position and repeat, taking a pace forward with each squat for 15–20 repetitions.

Starting position and action
- Begin in a neutral stance with your feet shoulder-width apart and arms by your sides.
- Step forward one pace with your right leg and then follow immediately with your left leg to bring your feet parallel, shoulder-width apart.
- From this position squat down, bending both knees, and sit back to bring your thighs almost parallel to the floor, raising your arms as you

Ex 8.28 Reverse lunges

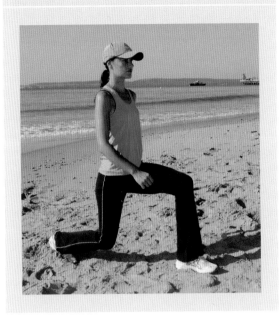

Starting position and action

- Stand upright with your feet together and then take a step back with your right leg.
- Flex your left leg and as your right foot touches the ground, bending both legs, lower down so that your right knee almost touches the sand and your left thigh is almost parallel with the floor.
- From this lowered position, drive through your left thigh and glutes to lift you back up to a standing position, bringing your right leg back to the start position.
- Repeat 15–20 times with your right leg lunging back before changing to your left.
- Note that it is your left thigh and glutes that are doing the work when your right leg moves and vice versa, as opposed to a normal forward lunge in which the leg that is stepping forwards is the one that is doing the most work.

Ex 8.29 Reverse lunge lift/jumps

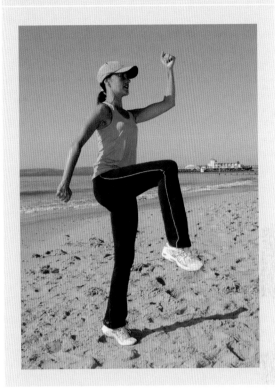

Starting position and action

- Perform this lunge as the reverse lunge, yet when you are driving up with your left leg you also lift the right leg that has just lunged behind you to bring the right thigh up in front, flexed at your hip and knee.
- To intensify this further you can develop this lunge/lift action to a lunge leap in which the force is substantially greater and you are pushing off your left leg with sufficient force to make a small jump as you drive your right thigh into the air. The lunge leap is a very challenging exercise and correct form should be maintained throughout.

Ex 8.30 Single-leg high step-ups

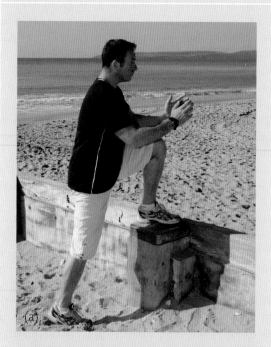

(a)

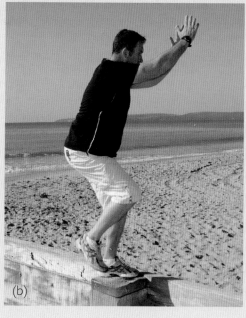

(b)

Starting position and action

- Stand next to a high wall or breakwater and lift your left leg to place your foot on the wall/breakwater.
- It is likely that your left knee will be flexed beyond a 90 degree angle.
- With your hands in front of you to assist balance, push through your left thigh and glutes to lift yourself up so that you are standing erect on the wall/breakwater.
- Then slowly bend your leg to lower you back to the sand under control before pushing back with your left thigh and glutes to repeat the action.
- Repeat 10–15 times.
- Then step back down with your left leg to the floor and repeat exercise, leading with your right leg.

Modification

- This exercise can be performed by standing sideways on or in front of the wall or breakwater and stepping up forwards, yet your balance is often compromised depending upon the height of the wall or breakwater you are stepping up onto.

Ex 8.31 Single-leg calf raises

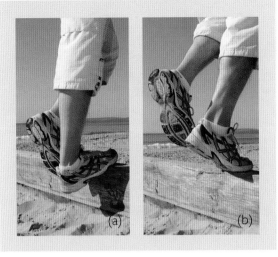
(a) (b)

Starting position and action
- Stand with your toes and forefeet on the edge of a step or rock, with your heels protruding back over the edge.
- Carefully take your weight on to your right leg and place your left foot at the back of your lower right leg.
- Slowly lower yourself down by allowing your bodyweight to act as the force pushing against the calf muscles of your right leg as you eccentrically contract them so that you are in a fully stretched position (of the calf muscle/gastrocnemius).
- Pause briefly and then concentrically contract your calf muscle and raise up on to your toes on the step to lift you up as high as you can (full contraction of the calf muscle).
- Aim for 15–25 repetitions before changing to your left leg.
- It is important to go through a full range of movement and to keep the movement slow throughout.

Ex 8.32 Bounding

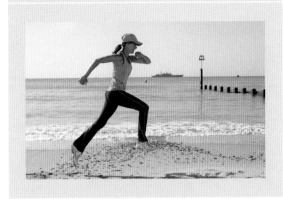

Starting position and action
- Find a flat area of compacted sand or grass. Pebbles will not be appropriate for this drill, nor would the promenade as it might be too hard.
- Begin by taking a few large strides to initiate the bounding technique then really try and push off the sand to maximise the distance of each bound.
- Ensure that with each foot 'landing' you are absorbing as much force as you can through your legs before pushing off again to leap on to the other leg.
- Repeat for 20–30 bounds on a suitable surface before walking back and repeating.
- Aim for 3–5 bounding sets.

Modifications
- Instead of bounding in a linear direction, try multi-direction bounding.
- Vary your direction to challenge your balance and proprioceptive skills, but be aware of your terrain, as this exercise can be detrimental to your knees or ankles if not performed with control.

Ex 8.33 Split-lunge jumps

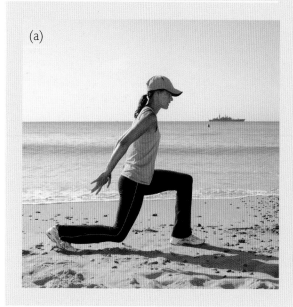

(a)

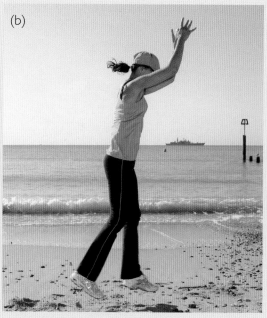

(b)

Starting position and action

- From a neutral stance, step forwards with your left leg into a lunge position, bending your left knee and lowering yourself down until your left thigh is parallel to the floor.
- As you lunge forwards make sure your right leg also bends so that your right knee almost touches the floor.
- In this position brace your abdominals and with your arms slightly bent, drive upwards pushing initially off your left leg then both legs to propel yourself into the air.
- Once in the air reverse your leg position so that you land with your right leg forwards and your left leg behind.
- As you land, cushion your landing by absorbing the force of gravity and decelerate the movement to lower yourself into the lunge position as before.

- In the lower position, drive up again with your legs to propel yourself into the air, reverse your leg position and then land with your left foot forwards and right leg behind.
- Repeat 20–30 times.

Modifications

- To intensify this exercise further, from the lunge position, drive yourself upwards to propel yourself into the air, but don't change legs. This way you are dynamically overloading one leg before working on the other.
- Aim for 10–15 repetitions on one leg before changing and repeating for another 10–15 repetitions.
- This exercise can be assisted with arm movement, when in the lower position – rapidly drive your arms upwards to assist the momentum of the exercise and help propel yourself into the air.

EXERCISES FOR ARMS

Ex 8.35 Breakwater dips

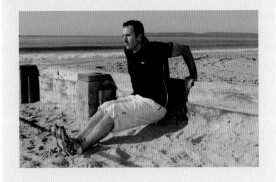

Ex 8.34 Concentration biceps curls

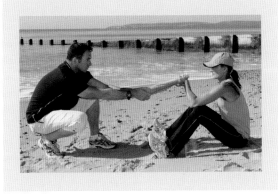

Starting position and action

- Sit down facing your partner with your knees bent and your elbows on your knees, holding both ends of a towel in your hands.
- Your partner should stand or sit in front and hold the centre of the towel with both hands to provide resistance.
- Keeping your torso still, curl the towel towards your shoulders keeping your elbows relatively still and on your knees.
- Your partner should apply resistance to the towel by pulling in the opposite direction.
- At full contraction, squeeze your biceps muscles, holding momentarily and then, still resisting your partner, return to the start position
- Keep your elbows positioned on your knees throughout, ensuring you return your arms to an almost straight position each time.
- Try not to lean back during the curl.
- Repeat 12–20 times.

Starting position and action

- Sit on a breakwater with your legs outstretched in front of you, with your feet on the ground and your hands on the breakwater, slightly wider than shoulder-width apart with your fingers pointing forwards.
- Lift yourself up to take your bodyweight on to your arms and, with your legs slightly bent, lower your torso down by bending your arms to almost 90 degrees with your elbows pointing behind you.
- From the flexed 90-degree position, push yourself back by straightening your arms to the start position with your bodyweight supported on your arms.
- Repeat 15–25 times.

Modifications

- To intensify the exercise, find a lower breakwater so that you are closer to the ground and more of your bodyweight is taken through your arms and shoulders.
- Alternatively, try placing your feet on a rock to raise them slightly, increasing the difficulty.

EXAMPLE BEACH WORKOUTS

Table 8.1		Cardio and resistance mixed circuit (1)		
Ex. no.	Page	Exercise	Repetitions	Option 1 circuit Complete all exercises in order
Warm-up	14–27	Warm-up variations (see chapter 3)		
8.4	89	Surf shuttles	30–45 sec	1/16
8.20	100	Gecko crawl with push-ups	15–20	2/17
8.24	103	Partner row	15–20	3/18
8.2	88	Breakwater up-and-over	30–45 sec	4/19
8.19	99	Kneeling partner-resisted chest presses	15–20	5/20
8.23	103	Back hyper-extension	15–20	6/21
8.33	110	Split lunge jumps	30–45 sec	7/22
8.26	105	Partner-resisted lateral raises	15–20	8/23
8.27	106	Squat walks	15–20	9/24
8.1	88	Breakwater hurdles	30–45 sec	10/25
8.9	93	Spiderman walk	15–25	11/26
8.32	109	Bounding	15–25	12/27
8.5	90	Burpees	30–45 sec	13/28
8.8	93	Slow eccentric abdominal curls	10–15	14/29
8.35	111	Breakwater dips	15–25	15/30
	237–40	Cool-down and stretch		

Table 8.2		Cardio and resistance mixed circuit (2)			
Ex. no.	**Page**	**Exercise** 15–25 repititions unless otherwise stated	**Option 1** **circuit** Complete all exercises in order	**Option 2** **super sets** Perform exercises alternately (A/B/C/D)	**Option 3** **giant sets/mini** **circuit** Perform these exercises in blocks in a circuit
Warm-up	14–27	Warm-up variations (see chapter 3)			
8.1	88	Breakwater hurdles (30 sec to 2 min)	A1/A12	A1/A3	A1/A6/A11
8.10	94	Horizontal balance	A2/A13	A2/A4	A2/A7/A12
8.5	90	Burpees (30 sec to 1 min)	A3/A14	Burpees	A3/A8/A13
8.18	98	Breakwater push-ups	A4/A15	B1/B3/ B5	A4/A9/A14
8.22	102	Railing pull-ups	A5/A16	B2/B4/B6	A5/A10/A15
8.3	89	Beach sprints (30 sec to 1 min)	A6/A17	Beach Sprints	B1/B7
8.25	104	Upright rows	A7/A18	C1/C3/C5	B2/B8
8.27	106	Squat walks	A8/A19	C2/C4/C6	B3/B9
8.17	97	Breakwater balance drills	A9/A20	Balance drill	B4/B10
8.34	111	Concentration biceps curls	A10/A21	D1/D3/D5	B5/B11
8.35	111	Breakwater dips	A11/A22	D2/D4/D6	B6/B12
	237–40	Cool-down and stretch			

PARK
WORKOUT

9

Whether you are simply going for a walk or a gentle jog to enjoy the open space free from cars and traffic pollution, or you intend to embark on a full-on fitness training session in the outdoors, maybe because you don't enjoy gyms or haven't joined one yet, a park is a fantastic place to exercise.

Working outside in a park environment often provides many more opportunities for exercise variation than you can get at home in your garden. For example, a park bench can be used to perform modified push-ups, dips, step-ups, squats or jumps. A low wall that rises as the path trails away is fantastic for changing both the nature and intensity of an exercise, due to the height differential. A simple log could provide a natural obstacle to jump over or hurdle, or even pick up and carry for 50m. Moreover, training in a park environment often brings out our inner child and it is quite easy to get carried away with an activity, such as leapfrog or tag, before realising how intense a bout of interval training you are undertaking.

To increase the potential of the park environment further, you could take a lightweight resistance tube or suspension cable along with you. Both are extremely portable and can be secured around posts, railings or trees to enable you to perform various resistance and suspended body-weight exercises. You could also mark out a running training area with small cones, twigs or apparel, while a medicine ball weighing 3–5kg is great to throw around and usually fits into a rucksack. If you are working with a personal trainer or, indeed, you are a personal trainer yourself, you might have an arsenal of portable fitness equipment in the boot of your car that is quick and easy to set up in an outdoor environment.

Whatever equipment you choose to use, safety should be paramount and the exercises you perform need to be effective and relative to your own fitness level. There is no point bursting a blood vessel in an attempt to perform a full pull-up, just because you have seen someone else 'rep' out 10 in succession before sprinting off to another area of the park as part of their own intense interval-training routine. Always look to modify the intensity of an exercise or even the exercise itself to suit your own fitness level and never attempt an activity without having an understanding of the potential risks or injuries relative to your own limitations.

I have not designed this chapter as a specific workout – it is a list of possible exercise options and variations to try in a park environment, collected loosely into various equipment options and muscle groups. In fact, as with other workouts in this book, the park workout can be supplemented with any of the exercises from the other workout chapters. The chapter concludes with several suggested workout plans for the park environment.

Ex 9.1 Step sprints

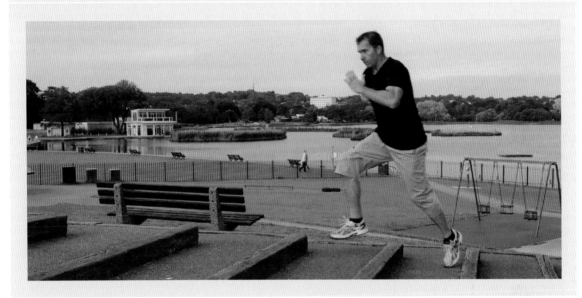

Starting position and action

- Start at the bottom of a long flight of steps, perhaps the steps on a tow path before a bridge, ideally with a minimum of 12 steps.
- Keeping your arms bent at right angles, and close to your torso, rapidly sprint up the steps one step at a time, aiming to 'pump' your arms in a rapid sprint action to sprint up as fast as possible.
- When you reach the top, turn around and walk back down to the start position.
- Repeat the step sprints 3–10 times depending on the number of steps in the flight and your own fitness level.

Modifications

- Take two steps each time as you race up the flight of stairs. By doing this your speed of stepping will be reduced slightly, yet you will need to push off more powerfully with your legs and glutes on each step. Your will need a more dynamic arm action to assist your stepping action.
- Again, on reaching the top, turn around, walk back down and repeat 3–10 times.
- This drill can be intensified again by stepping up three or four steps at a time, following the same repetition range as before.

OUTDOOR WORKOUTS

Ex 9.2 High-step knee lifts

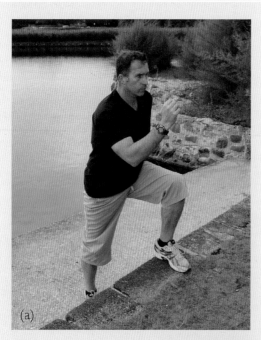

(a)

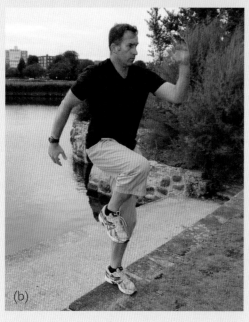

(b)

Starting position and action

- Stand in front of a relatively high wall, about 50–75cm in height.
- Place your left foot on to the high wall with your arms bent.
- Lean forwards slightly so that your weight is over your left leg.
- Drive your right knee upwards, pushing through your left thigh and glutes to lift yourself upwards, still with your weight on your left leg.
- As you step up, continue to drive your right knee upwards to touch your left hand at approximately hip height.
- Then lower your right foot back to the floor at a moderate pace, but under control.
- As soon as it touches the floor, drive upwards again with your right leg pushing through your left thigh and glutes.
- Repeat this knee driving/lifting action 15–30 times, before stepping down and changing legs, this time with your right leg on the wall and driving upwards with your left leg.

Ex 9.3 Rapid step-ups

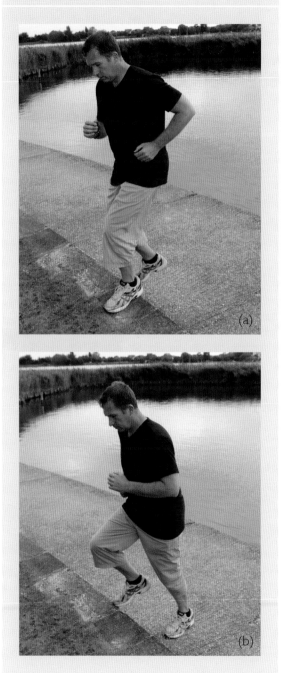

(a)

(b)

Starting position and action

- Start at the bottom of a set of steps or next to a low wall about 15–20cm high.
- Using the first step, step up and down with both feet (leading with your right leg) as fast as possible in sprint fashion until you have completed 50 steps.
- Use your arms to assist your 'running/stepping' action.
- Rest for 30 seconds to 1 minute and repeat, leading with your left leg.

EXERCISES FOR THE CORE

Ex 9.5 Suspended twisting crunches

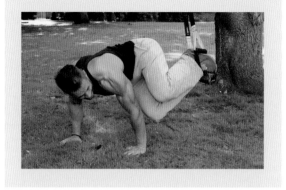

Ex 9.4 Suspended crunches

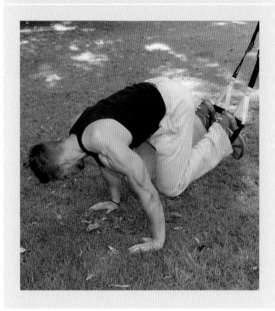

Starting position and action

- Sit on the ground as before, placing your feet into the stirrups and carefully roll over into a prone position with your hands on the ground.
- With your hands shoulder-width apart and arms slightly bent, brace your abdominals and flex at your hips and knees to draw your knees to your chest, but twisting each time to bring your knees alternately to the right side and left side in a twisting suspended crunch movement.
- Return to the start position, repeating for 20–30 crunch movements.

Modification

- A more intense modification is to perform the twisting crunch movement with your legs almost straight, in a 'pike' position.
- You will need to lift your hips as you twist and maintain tension through your core throughout.
- Slowly return your legs to the start position, but continue the movement, 'swinging' your legs to the left side, flexing at your hips to bring your legs towards your left shoulder.
- Repeat these 'pendulum swings' alternately to each side 15–20 times.

Starting position and action

- From a seated position, place your feet in the suspension cradles and rotate over to your right side to position yourself in a prone position on your hands, placed shoulder-width apart.
- With your feet in the cradles, brace your abdominals and bring your knees into your chest, engaging your abdominals, and then extend your legs, maintaining abdominal bracing throughout.
- Repeat 20–30 times.

Ex 9.6 Medicine ball power throws to floor

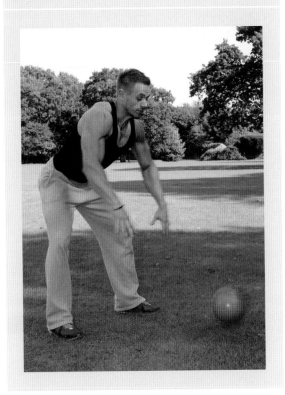

- Repeat for 10–15 power throws.
- This works well with a partner to take it in turns or pass the ball back to you.

Modifications
- This drill can be performed by modifying the throwing angle slightly, still aiming downwards, but targeting a point approximately 2–3m away to the side.
- Recreate a skiing action by throwing the ball slightly behind you, to your left then right.

Starting position and action
- Stand holding the medicine ball overhead with both hands. Your knees should be slightly bent, with your abdominals braced.
- Prior to throwing the medicine ball, tense your core muscles strongly before throwing the ball powerfully to the floor.
- Aim for the ball to bounce approximately 1m away from your feet, with partial flexion of your torso and a powerful arm action. The power emphasis of this movement initiates from the trunk, and not the arms.
- This is a rapid action and requires appropriate bracing to apply the force necessary.

Ex 9.7 Kneeling oblique throws

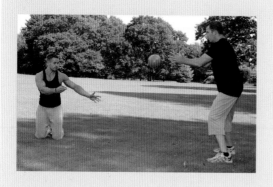

Starting position and action

- Kneel down on the ground, holding the medicine ball at arms' length, with your partner standing 3–5m away.
- Keep your hips in neutral and brace your abdominals as you rotate through the waist to throw the medicine diagonally towards your partner.
- When your partner catches the ball they should throw it hard to your other side for you to catch and absorb the force before twisting again at the waist to launch the medicine ball back to them.
- Don't allow unnecessary hip involvement or use the arms too much – the force should come from your torso.
- Remember not to lock your arms when holding the ball but keep them slightly bent.

Modifications

- This drill can be carried out 2–3m away from a brick wall. if you don't have a partner
- Both versions can be performed standing up, mimicking the rotational movements in tennis shots.

Ex 9.8 Reverse overhead throws

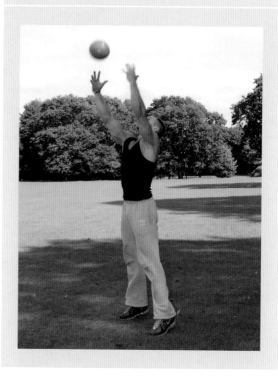

Starting position and action

- Stand with your feet shoulder-width apart holding a medicine ball at waist height.
- Brace your abdominals as you bend your knees and lean forwards slightly, swinging the medicine ball through your legs.
- Then extend your legs and back using your arms to help swing the medicine ball upwards to throw the ball forcefully into the air to land somewhere behind you.
- After the ball has come down to the ground, retrieve it and repeat.
- Make the movement dynamic, but keep it under control and begin with a relatively light resistance, building up to a heavier medicine ball over time.

Ex **9.9** Goalkeeper drills

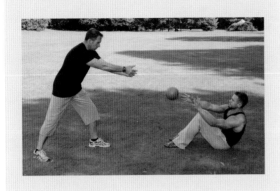

Starting position and action
- Lie face up on the ground with your knees slightly bent.
- You partner should stand 1–2m in front of you and hold a medicine ball.
- Perform an abdominal curl. At the top position, your partner should throw the medicine ball to your side, causing you to twist slightly as you catch the ball.
- As you catch the medicine ball you need to momentarily tense or brace to absorb the force.
- Throw the ball straight back to your partner before lowering yourself back to the floor and then repeat the curl-up, ready to catch again.
- Your partner should throw the ball so you have to reach to either side alternately, but make sure the timing is correct so that you always catch in the upper position and not while lying on the ground.

Modification
- Use a lighter medicine ball or even a football initially, and gradually work up to a heavier resistance over time.

Ex **9.10** Single-leg balances with lateral flexion

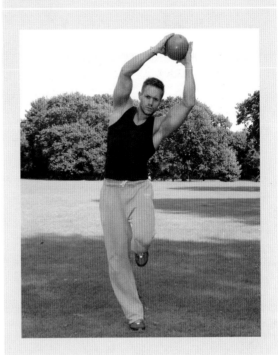

Starting position and action
- Hold a medicine ball overhead with both hands and take your weight on to your left leg.
- Keep your left leg slightly bent and lean across to your right side.
- Pause for 5 seconds, maintaining correct abdominal tension to ensure your core is braced, before returning back to a 'near neutral stance' with the medicine ball overhead.
- Repeat the exercise, this time leaning across to your left side, while maintaining balance and correct abdominal bracing, and pause for 5 seconds before returning to the start position.
- Repeat 10–15 times each side before lowering the medicine ball to the floor.

Ex 9.11 Abdominal curls to stand

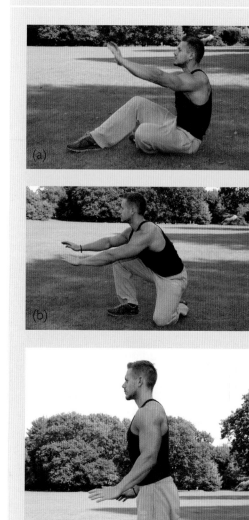

(a)

(b)

(c)

Starting position and action

- Lie down on the floor, face up with your hands behind your head and your knees bent.
- Dynamically curl up from your torso lifting your shoulders and upper back off the floor.
- As you continue to curl up into a sitting position, move your arms out in front of you, drop your left knee to the floor to allow you to carry on curling forwards but move your weight over your left knee in a split kneeling position with your left knee and shin on the floor.
- Push through your right thigh and glutes to stand up, bringing your left knee up and push yourself up to a standing position with your left leg now assisting.
- Bring both legs together, still with your hands out in front of you, and then reverse the movement to return slowly back to the floor.
- As you lower back to a kneeling position and then a sitting position, keep your movements under control and then slowly, in a curl movement, lower down to lie back on the floor.
- Repeat entire movement 3–10 times.

Modifications

- While it is likely that you will find preference to always drop the same knee to the floor, try and alternate your legs so that you vary the leg that you push up from each time.
- It is important that you don't just rely on momentum to lift yourself up or down. Try and maintain control and balance throughout all stages of this demanding exercise.
- If it proves too difficult with hands behind your head, keep them forwards to reduce the intensity.

EXERCISES FOR THE CHEST

Ex 9.12 Suspended chest presses

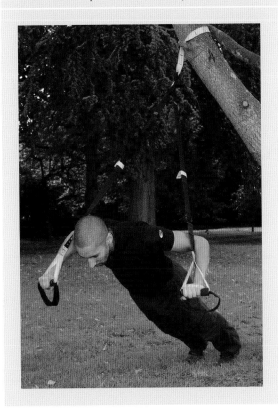

Starting position and action
- Hold both handles of the Suspension Training® system at chest height and face away from the anchor point so that as you lean forwards, your extended arms support your bodyweight, while keeping your abdominals braced to maintain rigidity through your torso.
- In this position, stabilise your shoulders and separate your arms by bending your elbows to lower yourself down so that your chest becomes level with your hands.

- Keep your abdominals braced to ensure correct spinal alignment and press through the grips to take you back to the start position.
- Repeat 10–20 times.

Modifications
- To intensify this exercise, walk your feet further back so that you are supporting more bodyweight when in the start position.
- To intensify further, lower the handles on the cables and place your legs further behind you so that your body is flatter to the ground and perform the press-up movement, keeping your core muscles and shoulder-complex muscles stabilised.
- This exercise can be intensified even further by elevating your feet on to a medicine ball, stability ball or bench.
- Perform the chest press with one leg raised off the floor to place greater demands on your core stabilisation muscles.
- Avoid dropping your hips to one side to compensate the rotational forces involved and maintain a neutral position and correct spinal alignment with correct core tension.

Ex 9.13 Push-up to stand-up drills

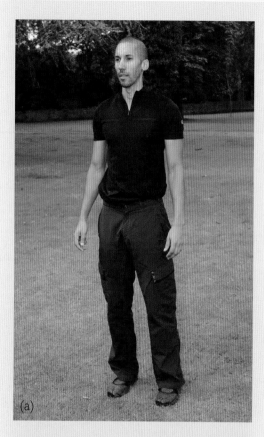

(a)

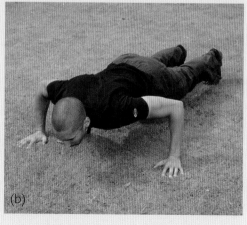

(b)

Starting position and action

- Start standing in a neutral stance with feet together or hip-distance apart.
- Bend your knees to squat down and then place your hands on the floor and walk yourself forwards on your hands into a push-up position, with legs outstretched behind you.
- In the prone push-up position, keeping your abdominals braced, bend your arms to lower your body to the floor. Then extend your arms, keeping your body rigid to return to the extended arm position.
- In this push-up position, push off your toes, drawing your knees towards your chest as in a squat-thrust action, to bring your knees under your chest, with your feet together.
- Push back with your arms to take your bodyweight on to your feet and then stand up straight, pushing off through your legs and glutes.
- From the standing position, repeat the push-up drill, this time performing two push-ups in the lower position before bringing your knees in and standing up again.
- Repeat these push-up to stand-up movements increasing your push-up counts each time, i.e. one push-up to stand up, two push-ups to stand up, etc.
- Aim for five total repetitions, eventually building up to ten or above.

Ex 9.14 Dynamic medicine ball push-ups

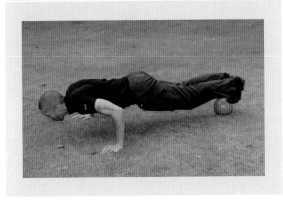

Ex 9.15 Chest presses using resistance tube

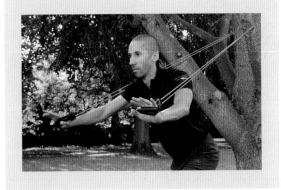

Starting position and action

- Start in a push-up position, with arms extended and abdominals braced.
- Place your feet on to a medicine ball and maintain your balance, keeping correct body alignment throughout.
- Bending at your elbows, lower your chest towards the floor and then extend your arms to return to the start position to complete a full push-up.
- Repeat 10–20 times, aiming to maintain correct form and control throughout.

Starting position and action

- Stand holding the handles of a resistance tube in each hand, with each tube secured or anchored around a post or tree behind you.
- Face away from the anchor point, with your hands by your shoulders, palms down and your elbows pointing behind you.
- Brace your abdominals and stand in a staggered stance, taking the tension up on the resistance tubes, and then extend your arms, pressing the handles forward so that they meet together with your arms extended.
- Pause briefly in this extended position and then slowly and under control return back to the start position with the handles by your chest.
- Do 15–20 repetitions, or repeat until fatigued.

Modifications

- Perform in a neutral stance, but ensure that you have appropriate core tension to maintain alignment as the elasticity of the stretched tubes will try to pull you backwards.
- To intensify further, try standing on one leg or perform the exercise from a kneeling position.

Ex 9.16 Medicine ball chest passes

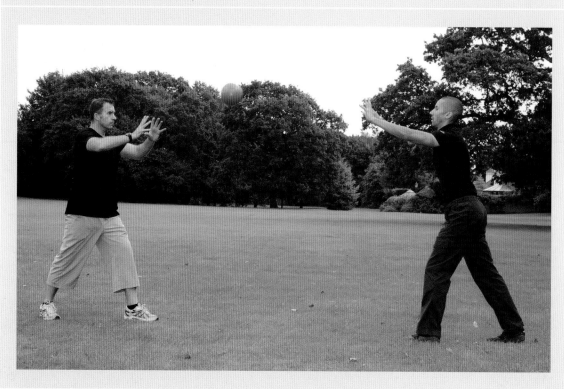

Starting position and action

- Stand in a neutral or split-stance, holding a medicine ball at chest height, with your partner opposite you, about 5–8m away.
- Brace your abdominals before you pass the medicine ball and rapidly push the ball away from your chest, keeping your upper body relatively still, towards your partner for them to catch it.
- Ideally stand so that you can 'chest pass' the medicine ball so that your partner can catch it at chest height.
- Your partner then returns the medicine ball in a similar forceful chest-pass action.
- Do 15–20 repetitions.

Modifications

- As you progress, take a step back to increase the distance between you and your partner, while still aiming to pass the ball at chest height accurately.
- This drill can also be performed standing opposite a wall if no partner is available.
- Instead of a chest pass, the medicine ball can be pushed to the floor in a similar technique to create a bounce pass. You will probably need to stand a little closer to your partner for this.

EXERCISES FOR THE BACK

Ex 9.17 Squat and rows

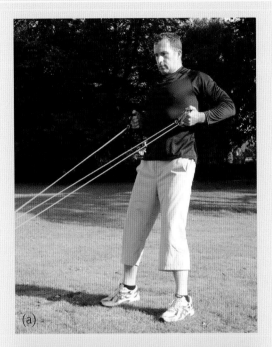

(a)

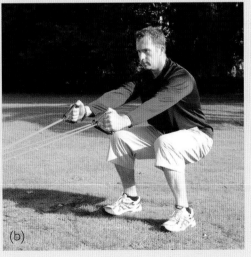

(b)

Starting position and action

- Wrap a resistance tube around a post, railing or tree and hold on to the grips.
- Keep your abdominals braced and lean back slightly while maintaining tension within the tube.
- Pull your arms back, retracting your shoulder blades and keeping your palms upwards, to bring your elbows back beyond your ribs.
- As you pull back on the handles, flex through your knees and hips to squat down and slightly backwards, to sit into a squat-and-row position with the resistance tube pulled in towards your ribs.
- Pause briefly in this position before standing back up and returning the handles to the start position.
- Repeat the row and squat movement 15–20 times.

Ex 9.18 Suspended back rows

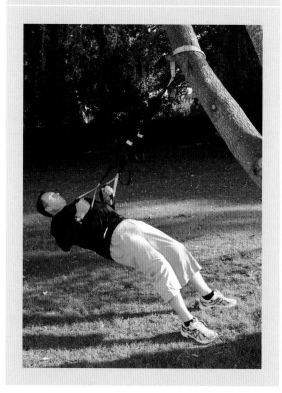

- On full contraction, with your chest level with the handles, pause briefly before lowering your torso back to the start position, with arms extended.
- It is important not to lose rigidity in your torso.
- Do 12–20 repetitions.

Modifications
- To increase the intensity, walk your feet further away so that you are at a lower angle and you are supporting more of your bodyweight.
- For a real challenge, place your feet on a raised bench, medicine ball, BOSU or stability ball.

Starting position and action
- Hold the grips at arms' length, facing the anchor point, and lean back, keeping your body straight and in alignment.
- Pull on the grips to bring your body towards the handles with either a palms-up, palms-inwards or palms-down grip.
- Your hand position will slightly affect the nature of arm movement and you should retract your shoulder blades and pull from your elbows, keeping the pulling action constant to keep the emphasis on your back muscles, maintaining a rigid body throughout the movement.

Ex 9.19 Seated alternate pull-downs

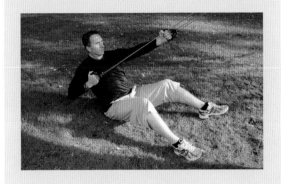

Starting position and action

- Sit down on the ground, holding the handles of two resistance tubes (two handles in each hand) with the tubes wrapped around a tree branch or secure anchor point above you.
- Lean back slightly, keeping your knees bent with your feet on the floor and your abdominals braced, and pull down with your right arm.
- Bring the handle down by contracting your back and biceps muscles to pull the resistance tube handles to approximately chest or shoulder height, with your elbow behind you.
- Hold this position briefly before returning the handles to the start position and then repeat on the other side by pulling down with your left hand to bring the handles of the other resistance tube to your left shoulder.
- Repeat alternate pull-downs for 15–30 repetitions.

Modification

- This exercise can be performed by working both arms together in a conventional pull-down technique.

Ex 9.20 Standing single-arm pulls

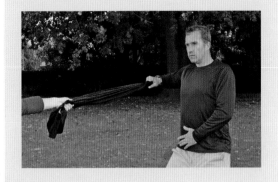

Starting position and action

- Stand facing your partner with your feet either in a neutral stance or a split-stance, holding a towel in your right arm at chest height with your arm extended.
- Keeping your legs slightly bent with abdominals braced, lean back slightly to control the tension of the towel.
- With your partner holding the other end of the towel and providing sufficient resistance, pull the towel towards you, retracting your shoulder blades and pulling back from your elbow, bringing your hand almost level with your chest.
- If in a split-stance, have your left foot forwards when pulling with your right hand and vice versa.
- Repeat 12–15 times on each side.

Modification

- This exercise can be performed as a dual workout whereby both partners are training their back in mirror fashion.

EXERCISES FOR SHOULDERS

Ex 9.21 Step-up with overhead presses

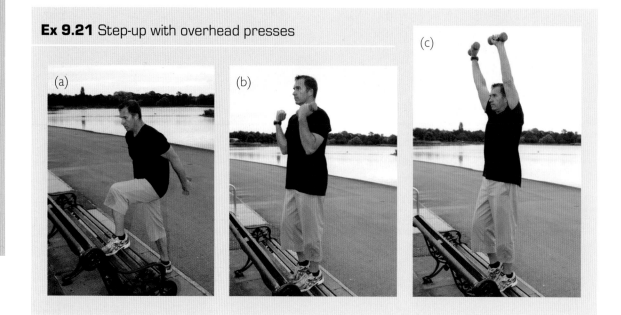

(a) (b) (c)

Starting position and action

- Stand behind a bench or step holding dumbbells in each hand with arms by your sides.
- Keep your abdominals braced and step up with your left leg on to the bench.
- As you push off this leg, to bring you up to a standing position on the bench with both legs, curl the dumbbells towards your shoulders, keeping your palms upwards.
- As soon as the dumbbells reach your shoulders, push them upwards using your triceps and shoulders to press them overhead, rotating the dumbbells in your palm to face forwards by pronating your forearms whilst lifting and supporting the weights.
- Pause briefly in the overhead press position before lowering the weights back to shoulder height with your palms facing your chest, and then as you step back down with your right leg, lower the dumbbells back to waist height under control.
- Finally step back to the floor with your left leg.
- Repeat this step, curl and press action 8–12 times.

Modifications

- This exercise can be adapted by stepping up with just one dumbbell – on the same side as the lead leg.
- A further modification is to hold a single dumbbell overhead while performing the step-up. You can vary this by holding the dumbbell with the opposite arm to lead leg or the same arm.

Ex 9.22 Single-arm throws

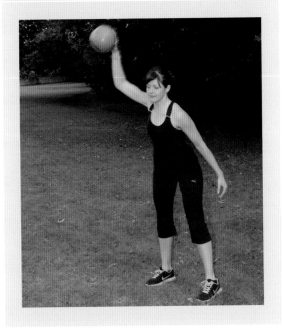

Ex 9.23 Reverse flyes

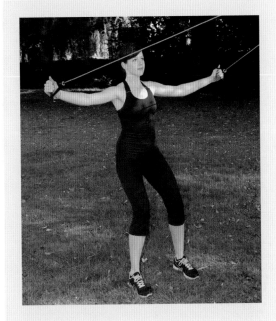

Starting position and action

- Stand holding a relatively light medicine ball (1–3kg) overhead in your right hand.
- Keeping your abdominals braced throughout, forcefully push down on the medicine ball, throwing the medicine ball towards the floor approximately 3–5m away.
- Repeat 6–10 times with one arm before using your other arm.

Modifications

- This drill can be performed using a bent – or straight-arm technique for variation and the direction and angle of throw can also be varied.

Starting position and action

- Wrap a resistance tube around a post or railing, holding on to the handles with your palms together.
- Keeping your knees slightly bent and your spine in neutral alignment, brace your abdominals and horizontally extend your shoulders, while keeping your arms slightly bent.
- Retract your shoulder blades as you bring your arms to a crucifix position, squeezing your rhomboid and posterior deltoid muscles.
- Hold briefly in this position before slowly returning the handles back to the start position.
- Repeat these reverse flye movements 15–20 times.

EXERCISES FOR LEGS

Ex 9.24 Suspension Training® squats

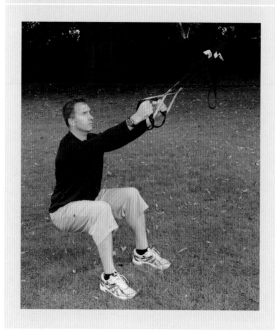

Ex 9.25 Suspension Training® squat jumps

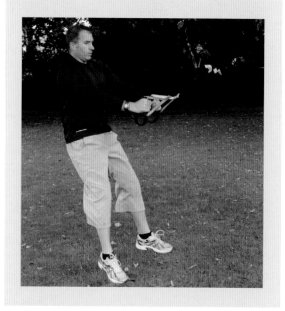

Starting position and action

- Attach the Suspension Training® system to an anchor point and hold on to the handles, facing the anchor point.
- With your feet approximately shoulder-width apart, lean back so that the cables support your weight and slowly bend your knees to sit back into the squat position, keeping your shins and torso parallel.
- Squat down until your thighs are parallel to the floor and then slowly extend your legs to return to the upright position.
- Repeat 15–20 times.

Starting position and action

- To intensify the squat, repeat the same process but add some power so that when you squat down slowly you forcefully push off through your legs to 'launch' yourself into the air and then 'cushion' your landing by bending your knees and squatting down again.
- When you push off you maintain your upper body position while holding the handles, keeping your arms flexed and shoulder stabilised and repeat for 10-15 repetitions..

Modification

- Perform the power-squat movement as before, but this time push off so that you land 1–2m to your left or right in a dynamic lateral squat.
- Lower back into the squat and repeat the lateral jump, returning to the start position.

Ex 9.26 Wall jumps

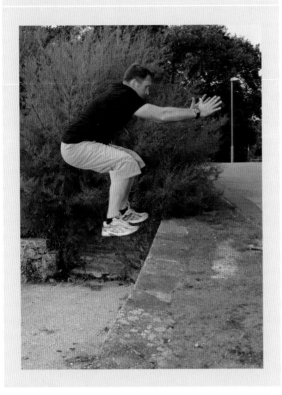

Ex 9.27 Path leaps

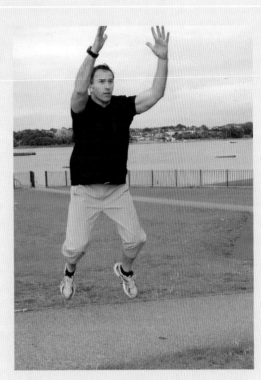

Starting position and action

- Stand in front of a bench or low-height wall with your knees slightly bent and arms by your sides and partially flexed.
- Squat down slightly and then push off, jumping up on to the bench/wall, flexing your knees and hips and driving upwards with your knees.
- Cushion your landing by bending your knees and squatting down, before pushing off to jump backwards off the bench/wall.
- As you land with your weight forwards, bend your knees and hips to absorb the force and lower into a part-squat position.
- Do 10–20 repetitions.

Starting position and action

- Find a path in the park about 1–2m wide and stand on the grass, facing across the path.
- With your feet hip-distance apart and knees bent, squat down and swing your arms forwards as you push off your legs, aiming to jump and land on the grass on the other side of the path.
- Cushion your landing by bending your legs to squat down and absorb your impact.
- After landing, stand back up and then turn around in preparation to repeat these horizontal path leaps.
- Repeat jump as before, for a total of 6–10 repetitions.

Ex 9.28 Leaf jumps

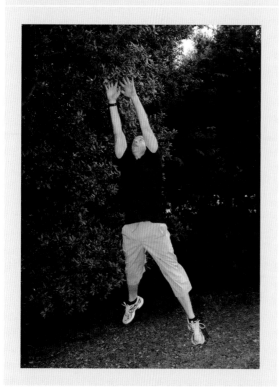

Ex 9.29 Squat jumps with floor touch and rotation*

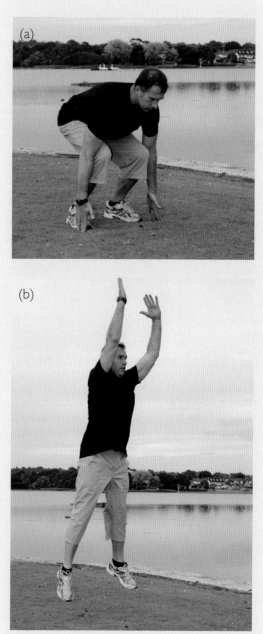

(a)

(b)

* Image shows modification

Starting position and action

* A variation of the path leap is to jump vertically and try and touch a leaf or branch.
* In a 'ready' position, with your knees slightly bent, push off through your legs and glutes to jump up as high as you can to reach the leaf or branch.
* This is a powerful vertical jump, so aim to repeat near maximal jumps 6–12 times before resting.
* The emphasis of this drill is not just to jump up lots of times but to really concentrate on a specific target and use maximal force to reach it.

Starting position and action

- Stand with your feet approximately shoulder-width apart in a neutral or slightly staggered stance.
- Bend your knees and squat down by 'sitting' back to bring your thighs almost parallel to the floor, keeping your upper body relatively upright.
- At the lowest part of the squat, reach down with both hands to touch the floor before dynamically pushing off through your legs and glutes to jump into the air.
- As you jump, aim to turn 180 degrees to face the other direction, and immediately as you land, bend your knees again to begin lowering yourself into the squat position.
- Repeat these squat-rotation jumps, touching the floor each time with both hands, 10–20 times alternately clockwise and then anti-clockwise.

Modifications

- If the squat with floor touch and rotational jump is too challenging, you could remove the turning element and stay facing the same way to make this exercise easier.

Ex 9.30 Partner-assisted single-leg squats

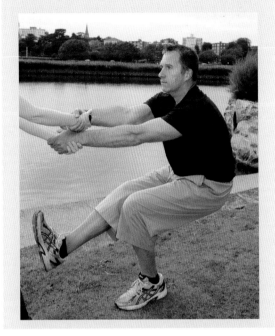

Starting position and action

- Stand upright with your feet together. Hold on to your partner's hands as you lean back so that your partner takes your weight.
- From this position, raise your right leg slightly, with your knee bent.
- Keeping a fairly upright stance while holding on to your partner's hands, bend your left leg to sit down into a squat position, keeping your right leg raised off the floor.
- Lower down until your left thigh is nearly parallel to the floor, pausing briefly before extending your leg, contracting your quads and glutes to return to the single-leg standing position.
- Repeat 10–15 times before changing legs and repeating on your right leg.

EXERCISES FOR ARMS

Ex 9.31 Suspended biceps curls

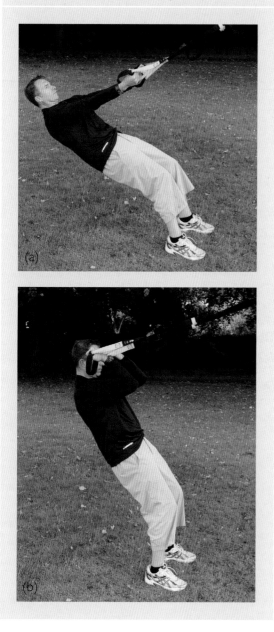

(a)

(b)

Starting position and action

- Stand facing the anchor point and holding both grips of the cables with your arms extended, palms up.
- Keep your body and torso rigid as you lean back to take your bodyweight through your arms, shoulders and back.
- Keep your elbows relatively still and curl your arms, bringing the grips towards your shoulders, maintaining abdominal tension and a rigid torso throughout.
- As you curl, your body will be pulled away from the floor and in the direction of the anchor point until you reach full flexion of your arms.
- Pause briefly in this fully flexed position and then slowly return your arms to the start position, controlling your bodyweight and keeping your elbows still.
- Repeat biceps curls 12–20 times.

Modification

- If you are struggling to perform more than two or three curls in strict form, walk your feet back slightly so that less of your bodyweight is taken through your arms.
- It is important not to move your elbow position – if you lower your elbows the exercise becomes more of a row technique and changes the emphasis from your biceps to your back and biceps.

Ex 9.32 Suspended triceps extensions

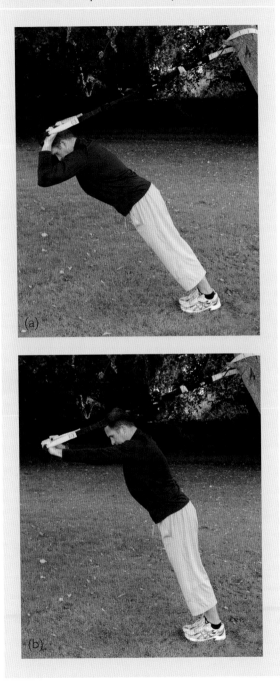

(a)

(b)

Starting position and action

- Stand facing away from the anchor point, holding the grips in both hands with your arms above your head.
- Brace your abdominals and lean forward, while maintaining a straight torso and correct body alignment, allowing your arms to bend with your palms facing upwards in the flexed position.
- In this flexed-arm position, keep your elbows fixed and contract your triceps to extend your arms back over your head, so that your palms are facing the floor in full extension.
- As you extend your arms your body will be pushed in the direction of the anchor point behind you, as you lift away from the floor.
- It is important not to have too much body-weight going through your arms, otherwise the exercise technique will be compromised.
- Maintain rigidity throughout this movement and don't compromise the movement by flexing at your hips to make the exercise easier if you are struggling. Instead, simply walk your feet forwards, so that you are supporting less of your bodyweight through your arms.
- Repeat 12–20 times.

Ex 9.33 Bench dips

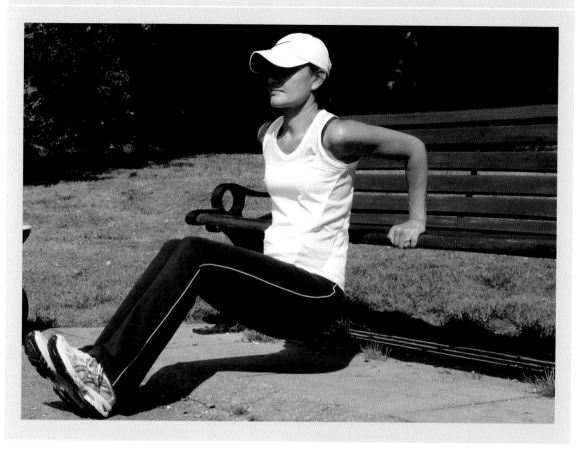

Starting position and action

- Begin sitting on a park bench and extend your legs out in front of you with your feet on the floor.
- Position your hands approximately shoulder-width apart on the bench, with fingers forwards.
- Lift yourself up, supporting your bodyweight on your hands and feet, with knees slightly bent.
- Slowly bend your arms to lower your torso towards the floor, bending your arms to almost

90 degrees at your elbows and keeping your elbows pointing behind you.

- From this position extend your arms to push you back to the starting position with your arms extended and your bodyweight supported through your arms, shoulders and legs.
- To make this easier, move your feet closer to the bench and bend your legs.
- Repeat 15–25 times, ensuring that you keep your weight over your arms, and do not allow yourself to tip forwards so that your legs take more of your bodyweight.

EXAMPLE PARK WORKOUTS

Table 9.1		Cardio and body-resistance mixed circuit		
Ex no.	**Page**	**Exercise**	**Repetitions**	**Circuit**
Warm-up	14–27	Warm-up variations (see chapter 3)		
8.5	90	Burpees	30–45 sec	1/16
9.12	123	Suspended chest presses	15–25	2/17
9.18	128	Suspended back rows	15–25	3/18
7.15	67	Commando crawls	20–30m	4/19
7.32	130	Step-up with overhead press	15–20	5/20
9.30	135	Partner assisted single-leg squats	15–20	6/21
9.11	122	Abdominal curls to stand	5–10	7/22
9.13	124	Push-up to stand-up drill	5–10	8/23
9.25	132	Suspension Training® squat jumps	5–10	9/24
7.4	59	Squat thrusts	30–45 sec	10/25
9.4	118	Suspended crunches	15–25	11/26
9.16	126	Medicine ball chest passes	15–25	12/27
8.28	107	Reverse lunges	15–25	13/28
9.31	136	Suspended biceps curls	10–15	14/29
9.32	137	Suspended triceps extensions	15–25	15/30
	237–40	Cool-down and stretch		

		Table 9.2	Alternate super-set/giant-set circuit options		

Ex no.	Page	Exercise	Option 1 circuit Complete all exercises in order	Option 2 super-sets Perform exercises Alternately (A/B/C/D/E)	Option 3 giant sets/ mini circuit Perform these exercises 2–3 times in blocks in a circuit
Warm-up	14–27	Warm-up variations (see chapter 3)			
9.14	125	Dynamic medicine ball push-ups	A1/A15	A1/A4	A1/A6/A11
9.20	129	Standing single arm pulls	A2/A16	A2/A5	A2/A7/A12
9.9	121	Goalkeeper drills	A3/A17	A3/A6	A3/A8/A13
9.29	134	Squat jumps with floor touch and rotation	A4/A18	B1/B3/B5	A4/A9/A14
9.6	119	Medicine ball power throws to floor	A5/A19	B2/B4/B6	A5/A10/A15
9.1	115	Step sprints	A6/A20	Step sprints	B1/B7
9.13	124	Push-up to stand-up drills	A7/A21	C1/C3/C5	B2/B8
9.23	131	Reverse flyes	A8/A22	C2/C4/C6	B3/B9
9.27 9.28	133 134	Path leaps/leaf jumps	A9/A23	Leaps/jumps	B4/B10
9.22	131	Single-arm throws	A10/A24	D1/D3/D5	B5/B11
9.26	133	Wall jumps	A11/A25	D2/D4/D6	B6/B12
9.31	136	Suspended biceps curls	A12/A26	E1/E4	C1/C4/C7
9.2	116	High-step knee lifts	A13/A27	E2/E5	C2/C5/C8
9.33	138	Bench dips	A14/A28	E3/E6	C3/C6/C9
	237–40	Cool-down and stretch			

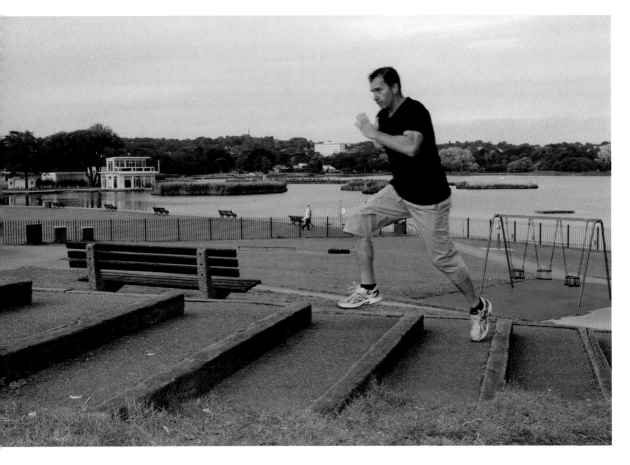

URBAN WORKOUTS

Urban workouts differ from park workouts in that the focus is on using minimal portable equipment, to utilise the environment around you. Whether you are sprinting up a flights of steps, using bridges, canal towpaths or even running up office-block fire escapes or multi-storey car park steps, remember not to confuse urban workouts with parkour or freerunning.

Urban workouts are of particular value if you have time in your lunch hour to exercise. Even a 15–20 minute exercise blast at lunchtime can be highly beneficial, as long as you warm up and cool down appropriately.

BOOTCAMP
// DRILLS

10

While 'bootcamps' originate from the hardcore training regime that marines and soldiers undertake during basic training, the term, thanks in large part to the media, has come to describe almost any activity involving a bit of effort to achieve results in a short time. From a purist's perspective, bootcamps seldom include equipment and the exercises are generally based on your own bodyweight and partner resistance. There are often team drills and physical challenges, which generate camaraderie, a sense of belonging and fun. Having taught numerous indoor and outdoor circuit classes throughout my career, I can certainly say that where there are partner-based and interactive drills, there is a greater deal of social interaction and retention.

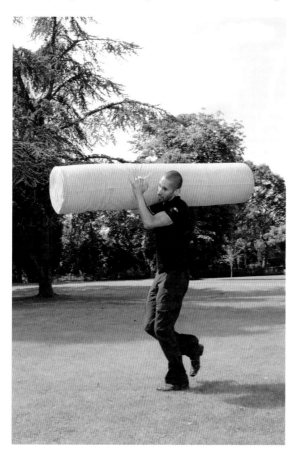

If you are considering joining a bootcamp class in a park near you, go and watch a session first to see if you like the instructor's style of teaching. A gung-ho/military style is not to everyone's taste, but if that is what you are after, British Military Fitness has been running bootcamps within the UK for over 15 years and all its instructors have a military background as well as being fully qualified trainers.

Regardless of the style of bootcamp or outdoor circuit workout, if signing up helps you to achieve your goals, then go for it. Alternatively, some of the exercises in this chapter might be of some value should you want to try your own bootcamp with a friend.

PARTNER DRILLS

Ex 10.1 Ball relays

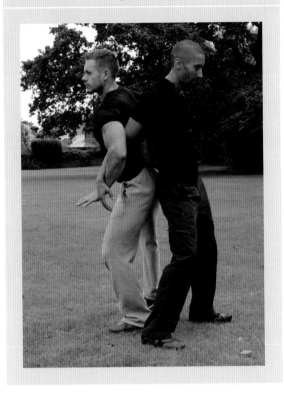

- Aim to carry the ball without dropping it and work in harmony with your partner, to achieve the distance in the fastest time, or racing against other opponent pairs.
- Depending upon the distance available and the number of players, this drill can be done as a relay or a single race, repeating carrying shuffles for up to one minute.

Modifications
- Carry the ball between your upper backs or indeed you could turn to face your partner and carry the ball between you, secured by pressing together at chest or abdomen height.

Starting position and action
- Set a target distance using a cone or other marker. Stand back-to-back with a partner of similar height.
- Place a ball in the small of your back and link arms to secure the ball in place (without touching the ball).
- Then, working with your partner, shuffle laterally towards the target, carrying the ball between you.

Ex 10.2 Escape drills

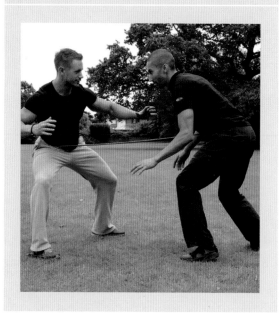

Starting position and action

- Tuck each end of a resistance tube loosely inside each person's shorts, T-shirt, etc.
- One person has to escape while the other has to stay as close as possible by 'marking them', using fast forward, backward and lateral foot movement and rapid direction changes to 'escape' from their partner.
- When the tube has stretched and then pops out of your partner's shorts, swap over and repeat drill.

Ex 10.3 Medicine ball reactions

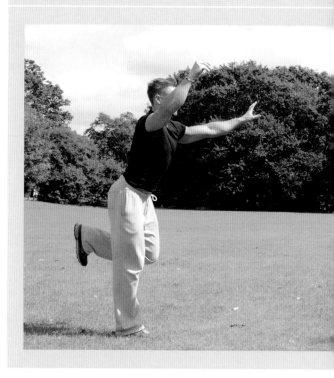

Starting position and action

- Stand on one leg with your abdominals braced and both knees slightly bent, holding a medicine ball.
- Facing a partner, throw the medicine ball to them without losing your balance.
- Your partner should catch the medicine ball (while also standing on one leg), absorbing its force, and then throw the ball back with force so that when you catch it you struggle to maintain your balance.
- Ensure that throughout the drill and especially when throwing and catching, your abdominals are fully braced and your legs are both slightly bent, and you remain standing on one leg throughout.

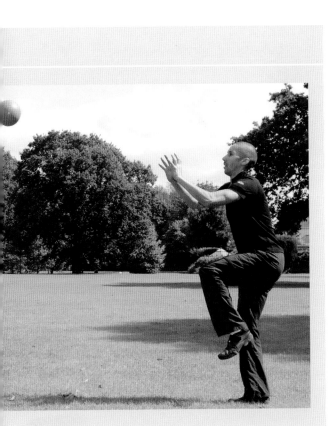

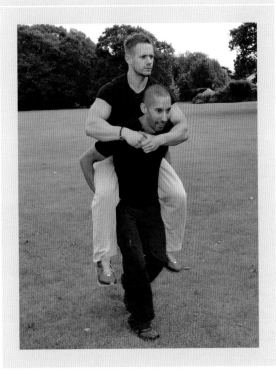

Ex 10.4 Piggy-back races

- Repeat for 30 seconds to 1 minute before resting briefly and repeating on your other leg (your partner should also change their balancing leg at this point).
- Repeat for 2–3 sets.
- It is important to keep your upper torso and legs relatively still to really challenge your proprioceptive balance and dynamic core stability.

Modifications

- If you do not have a partner, stand near a solid wall and bounce the medicine ball against it. Catch and repeat as before.
- Alternatively, to increase the balance element, try standing on a BOSU balance board.

Starting position and action

- This exercise is great for the leg muscles and for general fitness and requires you to brace your abdominals and torso in preparation for your partner to jump/climb on your back. Without the appropriate abdominal bracing and correct breathing during movement, this exercise can cause injuries if care and common sense aren't applied.
- Make sure that you can maintain your partner's weight in a relatively upright posture to avoid any discomfort or risk to your lower back.
- Aim to carry your partner over the required distance before swapping over so that your partner carries you back.

Ex 10.5 Leapfrogs

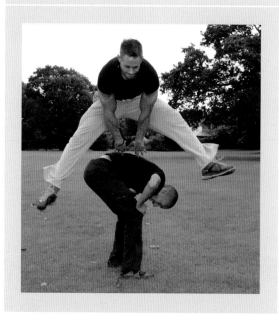

Ex 10.6 Wheelbarrow races

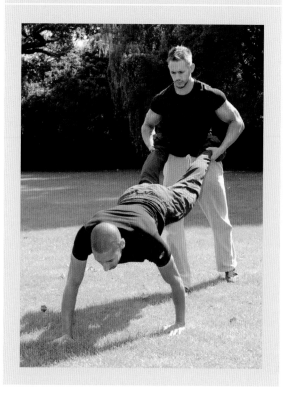

Starting position and action

- Your partner bends over and places their hands on their thighs or knees to support their torso as they tuck their head in, bending their legs slightly.
- Take a brief run up and place you hands on your partner's back, ready to push off your legs and their back to jump into the air, straddling your legs to jump over your partner.
- This exercise can be repeated in alternate fashion so that you leapfrog over each other to a desired distance or, alternatively, leapfrog over your partner and then crawl through your partner's legs.
- Make sure that as you go to jump over your partner you brace your abdominals to assist with the force required in the jump motion.
- In addition, when bending over waiting to be leapfrogged, you will need to brace your abdominals, torso and legs to avoid collapsing.

Starting position and action

- Start in the push-up position face down, supporting your bodyweight through your arms and shoulders with your legs behind you and feet together.
- Keep your abdominals braced to keep your body rigid throughout.
- Your partner then lifts your legs off the floor, holding on to your ankles.
- If you can maintain this elevated plank position, try and walk forwards on your hands over 5–10 metres, keeping your body and legs straight.

SPEED AND AGILITY DRILLS
ACCELERATION DRILLS

In addition to the fast-footwork ladder drills shown in chapter 4 (*see* pp. 34–38), further examples of acceleration and agility drills are shown below. These are great to mix into a workout either just after a couple of challenging leg drills or as a pre-exhaust to tire the legs before performing a challenging leg exercise.

Ex 10.7 Sprint starts

Starting position and action
- Start standing in a split-stance, leaning forwards ready to accelerate, with your arms bent and elbows by your sides.
- On the word 'go', drive forwards and upwards with your arms and legs to dynamically accelerate over a 5–10m distance.

- The emphasis of this drill is to focus on accelerating as quickly as possible over a relatively short distance.
- The important aspect is the first three to five steps that you take need to be really dynamic and forceful to drive the acceleration.
- On reaching the target distance, gradually decelerate to walking speed and then walk or jog back to the start.
- Repeat for 5–10 sprints.

Modification
- Lie face down on the ground with your arms bent and your hands on the ground next to your chest.
- On the word 'go', rapidly push yourself up by extending your arms and lifting your hips, to bring your feet into a sprinter's start (or set) position and then take your hands off the floor and lift your torso as you drive forwards with your legs to accelerate forwards.
- Take 5–15 strides forward, focussing on the first three to five steps of dynamic acceleration, pumping your arms and 'powering' forwards, working your legs and glutes.
- After the initial 10–15m acceleration sprint, decelerate over 10m to a walking pace, then turn around to face the other direction and lie down as before, with hands next to your chest facing the other way.
- Repeat for 5–10 sprints.

Ex **10.8** Cone drills

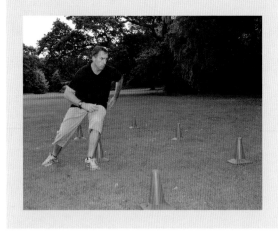

Starting position and action

- Position cones 3–5m apart, in a zigzag fashion (*see* fig. 10.1) and stand behind the cones at a 'start line' facing the cones.
- Lean forwards and then run in and out of the cones diagonally, but facing forwards throughout so that you shuffle/run to the right before changing direction and then shuffle/run to your left.
- Continue this zigzag movement in and out of the cones to the end and then turn around and jog back to the start.
- Repeat 5–10 times.

Figure 10.1 Set-up of cones for cone drills

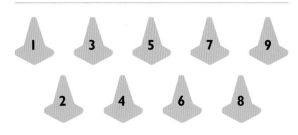

Ex **10.9** Shuttle runs

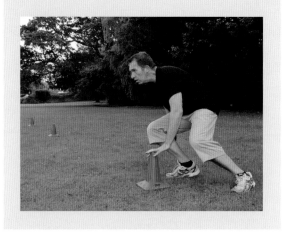

Starting position and action

- Position between three and six marker cones in a line approximately 3–5m apart.
- Then decide how you want to create the shuttle, as there are numerous variations.
- A classic variation is to run to the first cone and then as you reach it turn around and run back to the start position.
- Then run to the second cone and then back to the start followed by running to the third cone etc.
- Complete these shuttles until you have run to each cone and back again, then rest.
- This drill can be varied by running twice to each cone before moving on to the next, resting finally after running to the last cone twice and returning to the start.
- The sequence can be varied again by running to the furthest cone first, then back to the start, then running to the second furthest and back again etc.
- Another sequence variation is to combine these drills so that you run to cone 1 and back,

cone 2 and back, cone 3 and back all the way to the last cone, for example cone 6, and back, then to cone 5 and back, cone 4 and back, cone 3 and back, etc., all the way back to the start to finish and rest.

- You can also change the 'back position' that you run back to each time, for example, run to cone 1 and back to the start, then to cone 2 but then run back to cone 1, then run to cone 3 and back to cone 2, run to cone 4 and back to cone 3, etc.

- This drill can also be varied by running laterally, changing direction at each cone or even by facing the same way all the way through but running forwards and backwards to each relevant cone.

Modifications

- There are numerous cone drills that can be performed and the variations are almost endless. You can change the placement of the cones, the order or sequence you run between each cone and also the manner in which you move between the cones, either by lateral movements, running forwards or backwards, hopping, jumping, bounding, etc.

- You can then aim to touch the cone with your foot or hand as you reach it or even perform an exercise such as a push-up or squat-thrust at each cone.

Ex 10.10 Hill sprints

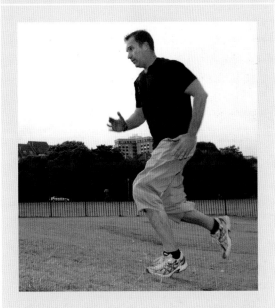

Starting position and action

- In a bootcamp environment, the length of hill sprints or gradient sprints will depend on what hills/gradients you have available and also the fitness of the participants involved.

- If you are working out on a recreation ground, there is the possibility that there is a mound of 'excess' earth or a bank on a relatively steep incline.

- If you are in the countryside and have the luxury of undulating hills and steep inclines then there is a lot more choice.

- If the hill or gradient is short (10–15m) then aim to repeat the sprint up 5–10 times.

- If the gradient is longer (30–100m) or shorter, but very steep, then aim to repeat 2–5 times.

OVERSPEED TRAINING

Overspeed training is a technique whereby you are either assisted or resisted in your running action, by gravity when running up or down varying hill gradients or through the use of bungee cords, pushing sleds or dragging car tyres, etc. For all overspeed training, whether running at speed down a gradient or using elastic ropes and training harnesses, correct form is vital and no compromise should be made for increased speed if the movement quality is diminished. The use of overspeed training encourages neurological adaptation within the muscles to deal with the faster movement mechanics due to the assistance of gravity (running down hill) or a bungee cord (assisted sprints).[22]

Wearing a resisted training harness, dragging a tyre/parachute, wearing weighted vests or running uphill create greater resistances on the muscles involved and thus these increased demands make you work harder and may assist you in recruiting more muscle fibres for the specific drill. Care should be taken not to overload the resistance too much if it compromises the movement either relative to a sporting application or if it compromises the technique unnecessarily.[23]

Ex 10.11 Bungee-cord-assisted sprints

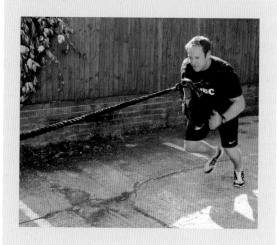

Starting position and action
- Wear a shoulder harness or a trunk belt that supports the bungee-cord system.
- Stand approximately 2–30m away from your partner (according to the length and elasticity of the bungee cord) with the bungee at full stretch.

- Facing your partner, stand in a sprint start or 'ready' position, poised to accelerate, with your arms bent.
- On the word 'go', drive forwards with alternate arms and push off your legs in a sprinting action towards your partner.
- As you begin to sprint, your partner pulls on the bungee cord, to keep the tension and elastic assistance throughout your sprint.
- The overspeed effect means you have to adjust your normal running action to deal with the added speed and this can lead to neural adaptations, the muscles experiencing a faster running action than normal.
- As you pass your partner, decelerate comfortably and then walk back to repeat.
- Repeat 3–8 times.

Modifications
- This exercise drill can be repeated by the same person before resting or you can swap places with your partner, repeating the sprint drill alternately for 5–10 sprints.

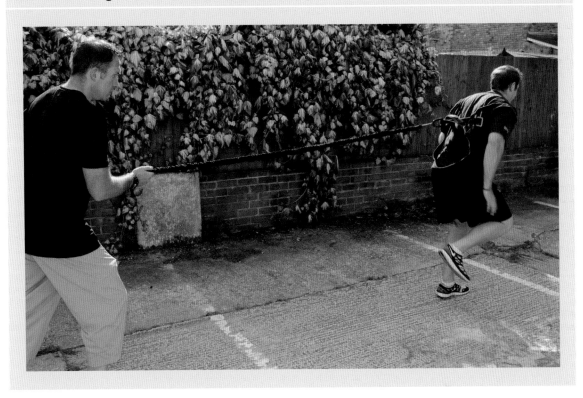

Starting position and action

- Wearing a trunk belt or shoulder harness with a bungee cord attached to the rear, work with a partner, who will follow your path across the field.
- Set yourself a distance of 50–75m to sprint, yet run against the increasing resistance of a bungee cord.
- Start in a split-stance in a sprint-ready position.
- Drive off, pushing through your legs and glutes and pumping your arms, with arms bent at 90 degrees to accelerate forwards against the resistance of the bungee.
- As you run forwards, your partner should follow you but at a slower speed to allow the resistance to get stronger, but over a greater distance than a static line will allow.
- Continue powering forwards over the distance and then gradually decelerate down to a walk before resting briefly then repeating.
- Depending upon your fitness level, aim for 5–10 repeated sprints over a 50–75m distance.

Modifications

- You can create an excellent resisted sprinting drill by dragging a tyre or running with a sports parachute behind you over a distance of 40–80m and, depending upon your fitness level and desired goal, repeating 3–5 times.

Ex 10.13 Cone co-ordination drills

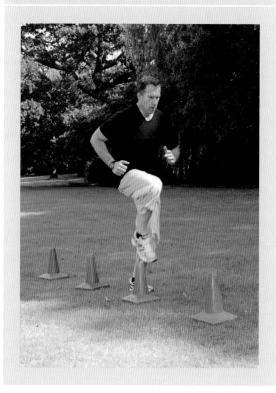

Ex 10.14 Cone jumps

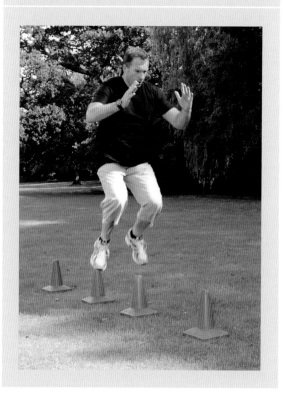

Starting position and action

- Line up the cones spaced about one stride length apart.
- Stand just to the left at the beginning of the cones in preparation to accelerate.
- The technique here is to have a rapid hip lift and placement with your right leg going over the cones and your left leg following just outside of the cones.
- Sprint-hurdle the line of cones before jogging back and repeating, this time with your left leg performing the sprint hurdle action with your right leg outside the line of hurdles.
- Repeat the co-ordination sprints 3–5 times on each side.

Starting position and action

- Position 6–10 cones in a line spaced approximately 1m apart and stand behind the cones, with your feet about shoulder-width apart, arms slightly bent and at your side.
- Bend your knees and lean forwards slightly before partially squatting down to jump over the first cone.
- As you jump, lift your knees over the cone and then extend your legs.
- Bend your knees to cushion your landing, but rapidly push back down with your legs to leap over the next cone, using your arms to assist your drive if necessary.

- Continue to jump repeatedly over each of the cones then walk back and rest before repeating for 5–8 complete sets.

Modifications: Plyometric jumps

- An alternative variation without hurdles is to jump diagonally to your right, then on landing jump to your left at a 75–90-degree angle.
- Repeat these diagonal jumps over the 10–20m distance before walking back and repeating 3–5 times.
- Aim for full power on each jump to achieve a near-maximum distance for each jump.

Ex 10.15 Lateral cone jumps

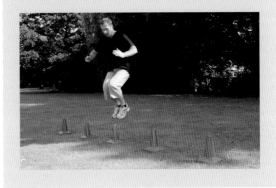

Starting position and action

- Place 10–15 cones (15–20cm high) along the floor, approximately 50cm apart.
- Stand at right angles to the first cone so that your left leg is next to the first cone.
- With feet hip-distance apart or closer, bend your knees and then drive up to jump over the cones in succession until you have completed the line.
- After completing the set of jumps, walk back, take a short rest and repeat, turning to face the other direction with your right foot closest to the cones.
- Do 3–5 sets on each side.

Modifications – Lateral cone jumps with rotation

- A variation of the above exercise is to jump over the cones yet rotate to face opposite directions after each landing, so that when jumping with your left leg closest to the cones, you turn 180 degrees in mid-air, to land with your right leg closest to the next cone.
- Continue to jump over the cones to the end, turning 180 degrees right and left on each jump.

TYRE DRILLS AND SLED PUSHING

Ex 10.16 Farmer's walk with spare tyres

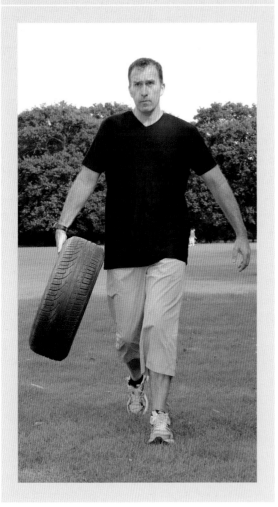

Starting position and action

- Place a car tyre on the floor next to your feet.
- Bend down and, keeping your abdominals braced and your torso fairly upright, take hold of the tyre by the rim and then extend your legs to return to the standing position, holding the tyre by your side.
- Maintain an upright stance with your abdominals braced throughout and walk forwards over a distance of 30–50m.
- Ensure you have your shoulders retracted, working your back and shoulder muscles while holding the tyre, and avoid leaning over to one side.
- After completing the desired distance either turn around and return or place the tyre on the floor and rest before returning.

Modifications

- If available, you can use two tyres, holding one in each hand.
- Another option is to hold the tyre above your head with one or both hands.

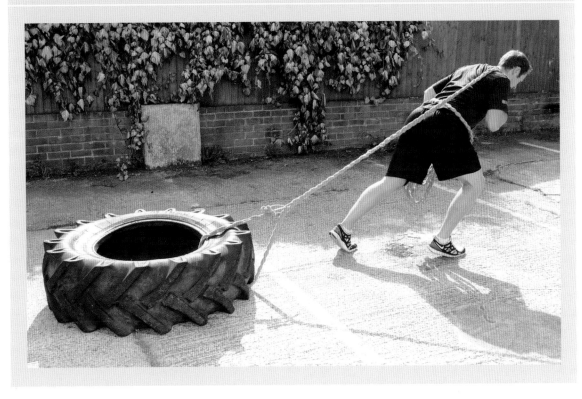

Starting position and action

- Ideally you will need a shoulder harness with a rope attached to the tyre on the ground behind you. If no harness is available, you can tie the rope loosely around your waist, but this will compromise the nature of movement slightly and change the forces throughout your body.
- Lean forward with one leg in front of the other to take up any slack on the rope.
- Then with abdominals braced, drive your arms and legs forwards to accelerate off, dragging the tyre behind you.
- Maintain abdominal tension to keep your torso stabilised as you drag the tyre across the ground, making sure you do not lean so far forward that you lose balance.
- Ensure you are driving powerfully with your arms and legs to maximise your acceleration.
- On completing the desired distance, step out of the harness and walk around to recover before refitting the harness and repeating back to the start position.

Modifications

- Obviously the size of the tyre chosen can vary according to your fitness level and bodyweight.
- Alternatively, to add intensity, strap two or more tyres together for a very advanced tyre drag.

Ex 10.18 Tyre flipping

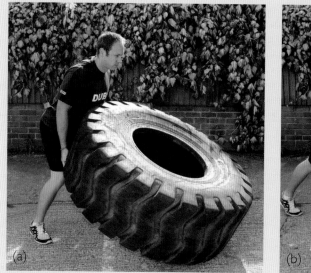
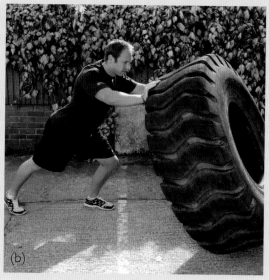
(a) (b)

Starting position and action

- For this drill you will need to use a tractor tyre as anything smaller will change your lifting technique and potentially cause you more back strain than if using a larger tyre.
- Position yourself behind the tractor tyre and squat down, bending your knees and keeping your back fairly straight. Place your hands under the edge of the tyre, with palms upwards and arms slightly bent.
- Keeping your abdominals braced, lift one side of the tyre up on to its opposite edge using your legs and glutes to initiate the lift. As you near a standing position while holding the tyre, use your arms to lift the tyre further so that your hands are near chest height.

- At this point, bend your legs slightly and 'flip' your hands around, so that you now hold on to the edge of the tyre facing downwards. This will allow you to change from a lifting technique to a pushing or 'flipping' technique.
- Continue to push with your legs and arms so that the tyre 'flips' over to the other side.
- When it has come to a rest, repeat the entire movement, squatting down and placing your hands under the edge of the tyre as before.
- Repeat the lifting, pushing and flipping technique to flip the tyre over a 10–20m distance.

Ex 10.19 Tyre pulling

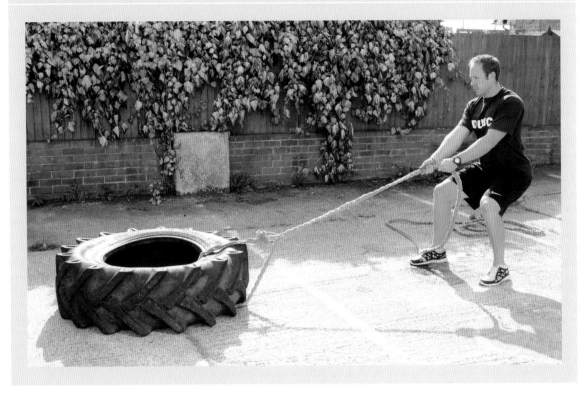

Starting position and action

- Tie a 20–30m length of rope around a tyre.
- For the standing pull, take hold of the rope, facing the tyre and take up any slack.
- From a split-stance position (one foot in front of the other), lean back holding the rope with your arms slightly bent.
- Keeping your abdominals braced, pull on the rope hand over hand to drag the tyre towards you.
- Use your back and arm muscles to pull the tyre, keeping your legs slightly bent and torso in a stabilised and braced position.
- For very heavy tyres you might need to use your legs and bodyweight more to assist your arms and back as you pull.

Modification

- This exercise can be performed sitting on the ground with your legs outstretched in front of you, performing the hand-over-hand technique to pull the tyre.

Ex 10.20 Tyre lifts/pull-downs

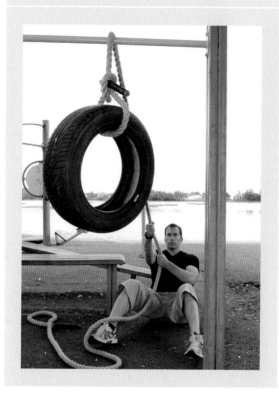

Starting position and action

- If there is an opportunity to secure a long rope to a tyre and throw it over a suitable tree branch or secure high bar, this is a fantastic way of training your back and arm muscles by pulling on the rope repeatedly according to the length of the rope, dragging the tyre with each pull.
- For this exercise you are limited by the length of rope you have, a suitable resistance – relative to your own strength – and finding a suitable high bar or tree branch that is safe and that you are allowed to use.
- Begin with a bar or tree branch ideally at least 2–3m in height.

- Tie the end of the rope to a car tyre or tyres to act as resistance.
- Sit down under the bar, with your legs wide to assist stabilisation.
- Begin to pull on the rope until the 'slack' of the rope has been taken up and then brace your abdominals in preparation for the strain of lifting the tyres.
- Pull down on the rope with your arms and in a hand-over-hand action that lifts the tyre/s off the floor.
- Depending upon the height of your bar/branch and also the length of rope you are using, you might find that it only takes 5–8 pulls before the tyres are at the top next to the bar/tree branch. When this happens, reverse your movement and lower the tyres back to the floor, slowly and under control.
- Repeat this lifting and lowering of the tyres for 30–60 seconds.

Modifications

- If you are lucky enough to have a very long rope, then instead of 'lifting' the tyres against gravity you can 'drag' the tyres across the ground, until they reach the bar/tree.
- At this point, lift the tyres up towards the bar and then lower as before.
- With this 'dragging' action you can really intensify the exercise by increasing your pulling speed and increasing the overall dynamic of the exercise.

Ex 10.21 Hitting tyre with sledgehammer

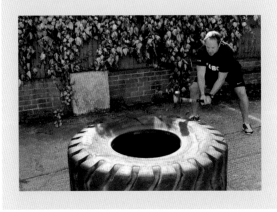

Ex 10.22 Sled pushing

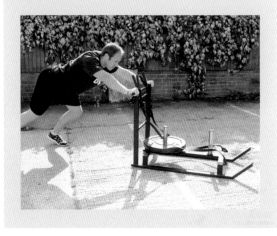

Starting position and action

- Ideally use a large tyre, such as a tractor tyre lying on its side.
- Stand upright holding a sledgehammer by its handle and then with your knees bent and abdominals braced, swing the sledgehammer in a downward action to strike the tyre with force.
- Ensure that you are not over-twisting when swinging the sledgehammer as this can cause injury.
- Begin with relatively small swings but over time, as your body and muscles adapt to the forces on the body, build to full overhead and diagonal rotations, not dissimilar to the old fairground challenge of hitting a sledgehammer on to a board to propel a ball upwards to ring a bell. This time there is no bell and you can have as many swings as you can handle.
- Begin with 20–30 seconds of striking the tyre, building up to one minute of repeated swings and strikes.

Starting position and action

- Some personal trainers and bootcamps have the use of a sled, which can be loaded with weights, car tyres or even people and is an excellent device for functional strength training.
- Load up the sled with suitable resistance so that it is moveable but with effort.
- Position yourself behind the sled, maintaining abdominal tension, and lean on to the sled in a split-stance position.
- Without holding your breath, aim to push the sled 20–30m across the grass before resting. The sled push should not exceed 30–40 seconds due to intensity.
- Rest for 1–2 minutes and repeat 2–3 times.

VIPR AND BOSU DRILLS

Ex 10.23 BOSU walk-downs

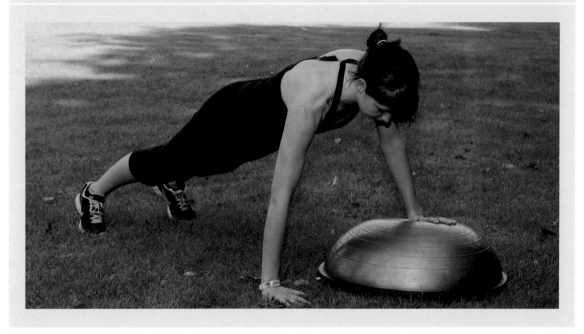

Starting position and action

- Begin in a prone position with legs out-stretched behind you and with your hands on a BOSU, approximately 20cm apart, keeping your abdominals braced and a rigid torso throughout.
- Carefully take your weight on to your left hand as you lift and place your right hand on to the floor, to the side of the BOSU.
- Then carefully move your left hand to the floor, adjacent to the BOSU.
- When both hands are supporting your body-weight on the floor, maintaining abdominal tension, lift your right hand and place it back on to the BOSU.

- Then bring your left hand back on to the BOSU into the starting position.
- Repeat 15–20 times.

Modifications

- To make this exercise easier, perform the movement on your knees.
- Alternatively, if the instability is too challenging, try separating your feet to a wide stance, or perform the movement off a low step.
- To intensify this movement, try lifting one foot into the air, or even add a press-up when your hands are in an asymmetric position, i.e. one hand on the BOSU and one hand on the floor.

Ex 10.24 BOSU split squats

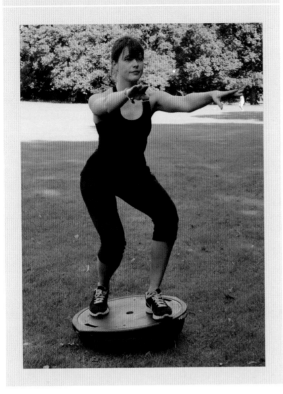

Starting position and action
- Stand in a split-stance position on the BOSU.
- Keeping your torso upright with your arms by your sides, squat down, maintaining abdominal bracing, as you sit back until your thighs are parallel to the floor.
- Pause briefly at the lowered position before standing back up, pushing off through your thighs and glutes to return to a standing position with your knees slightly bent.
- Repeat these split squats for 10–20 repetitions.

Modification: BOSU jumps
- To intensify this exercise and add a greater stabilisation requirement, from the split-stance squat position, as you stand up, dynamically push against the BOSU to launch you into the air before landing back on the BOSU and squatting down again.
- There are numerous variations of this BOSU jump, from changing your legs in mid-air to land with your other foot in front on the BOSU.
- Alternatively from a neutral stance, squat down partially with your knees before dynamically pushing off your legs to jump into the air then land back on to the BOSU in a balanced position, having rotated between 45 and 90 degrees.
- Jump from the floor to the BOSU or indeed from the BOSU to the floor or from one BOSU to another, maintaining your balance on each take-off and landing.

Ex 10.25 BOSU squat thrusts to balance

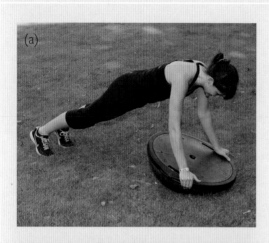

(a)

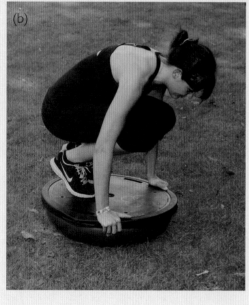

(b)

Starting position and action

- Hold on to a BOSU by its edges with both hands.
- Initially position your legs outstretched behind you, in a prone position as if to perform a push-up.
- From this position, with your abdominals braced, push off your toes, lifting your hips up, and bend your knees to draw them in so that your feet and knees come right underneath your chest and you 'land' on the BOSU in a crouched position.
- In this position, brace your abdominals again and push off your toes, lifting your hips up so that you can drive your legs back to the start position in a squat-thrust movement.
- Repeat squat thrusts 10–20 times.

Modifications

- Stand up after each 'jump-in', i.e. from the leg-extended position, push off to land both feet on to the BOSU and then stand up on the BOSU, maintaining your balance.
- Squat down again to grasp the edges of the BOSU with both hands and then, bracing your abdominals, push off with your legs to extend them back to the floor in a squat-thrust action.

Ex **10.26** BOSU dynamic lateral push-ups

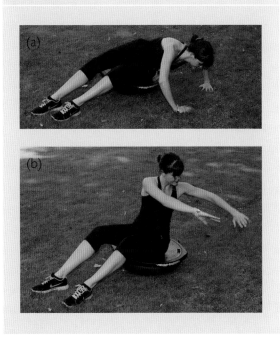

(a)

(b)

Ex **10.27** BOSU ViPR tilts

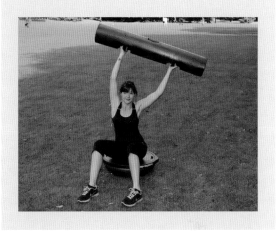

Starting position and action

- Sit on a BOSU (flat side up) with your knees slightly bent and feet together on the floor.
- Keep your abdominals braced and lean across to your right side. Bring both arms towards your chest and as you lose balance and 'fall' to the floor use your arms to decelerate your fall, in a lateral press-up action.
- As you lower, forcefully push back with your arms, shoulders and chest to an upright seated position.
- In this position, lean across to your left side so that you 'fall' across to your left, bringing your arms to the floor as before then dynamically pushing off the floor to return to the upright seated position.
- Repeat 8–12 times on each side.

Starting position and action

- Sit on the BOSU, flat side up, holding a ViPR above your head with your abdominals braced.
- Keep your feet together on the floor with your knees bent, and sitting centrally on the BOSU.
- Tilt the BOSU to the left and the right while maintaining your balance and keeping the ViPR over your head.
- Ensure you are bracing your abdominals throughout the movement, especially as you adjust your body position.

Modifications

- Instead of holding the ViPR over your head you can hold it at chest height, but ensure you use a lightweight ViPR. Alternatively, you could hold a medicine ball with both hands gripping the ball, either overhead or in front of your chest while bracing your abdominals and tilting the BOSU to either side.
- To increase the stabilisation requirement, place your feet either on a medicine ball or upturned BOSU (flat side down).

Ex 10.28 BOSU Russian twists

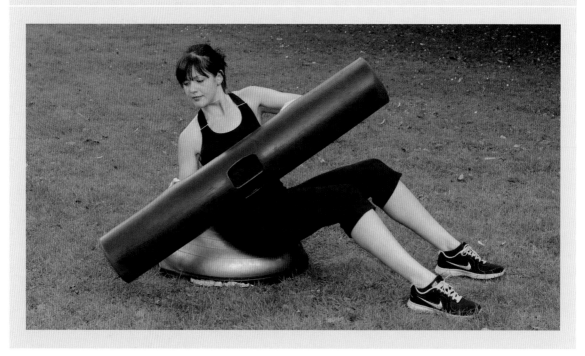

Starting position and action

- Sit on a BOSU with the flat side down, your feet on the floor, with your knees bent.
- Hold on to a ViPR or medicine ball with arms slightly bent held at chest height and lean back to almost a 45-degree angle, keeping your abdominals braced.
- Maintain this angle and rotate your torso to your right, holding the ViPR at arms' length, to touch the floor on your right.
- Then rotate back to your left, maintaining core tension and body angle to touch the ViPR tip to your left side and then rotate back to your right and continue rotations for 20–30 repetitions.
- Ensure you follow the path of the ViPR with your head to get full torso rotation, rather than just throwing your arms to the left and right.

Modification – BOSU Figure-8's

- Repeat the exercise above, again holding a ViPR or a medicine ball and instead of rotations to either side, perform a figure-8 movement to simulate the paddling action when canoeing/kayaking, keeping your abdominals braced and feet together on the floor.
- Repeat for 20–30 complete movements.
- To intensify the stabilisation requirement try placing your feet on a medicine ball.

Ex 10.29 ViPR cylindrical lifts

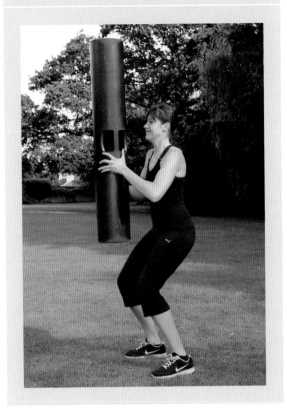

- Slowly squat down to repeat the movement, maintaining your grip on the ViPR as you lower, before driving back upwards from the squat position using your legs to power the ViPR up again before releasing your grip.
- As you 'catch' the ViPR your grip will be lower down the tube. Continue to work your way to the ViPR's base, maintaining neutral spine throughout all the lifts and keeping the ViPR vertical.

Modification

- To increase the stabilisation element, perform the cylindrical lift while standing on a BOSU.

Starting position and action

- Stand with your feet hip-distance apart and hold a ViPR upright on its end in front of you.
- Partially squat down and grasp the ViPR with both hands firmly, with elbows bent but fixed, while bracing your abdominals to maintain correct spinal alignment.
- Lift the ViPR in front of your chest, holding it upright, and bend your legs then forcefully extend to drive the ViPR upwards, essentially lifting it towards the ceiling.
- As you drive the ViPR upwards release your grip, allowing you to grip further down the base of the tube.

Ex 10.30 ViPR lateral flip drills

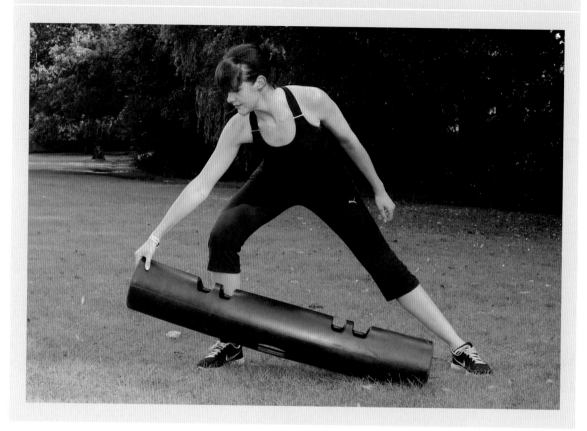

Starting position and action

- Take hold of the ViPR and tilt it to the right maintaining contact as you lower it to the floor.
- To ensure correct body positioning you will need to step to your right to maintain contact.
- Just before the ViPR touches the floor, lift it by its end, maintaining abdominal tension to flip it back through a vertical position to the other side.
- Transfer your hands to tilt the ViPR, continuing its direction of movement towards the floor on your left side.
- This time you will need to shuffle to your left.

- Before the ViPR touches the floor, lift it back (using your right hand) to the starting position and repeat, alternating right and left for 15–20 repetitions.

Modifications

- Use the opposite hand to control the ViPR as it lowers to the floor.
- Drop the ViPR to the floor before lifting it back to vertical.
- If there is space, 'flip' the ViPR continually to the right 5–10 times before flipping it back again to the left.

Ex 10.31 ViPR integrated clean and presses with lunge

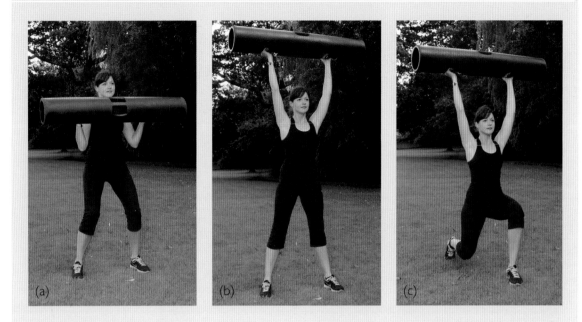

(a) (b) (c)

Starting position and action

- Brace your abdominals and, holding the ViPR by the handles, forcefully extend your hips and legs to lift it, initially to your chest (in a 'clean' action) before you 'press' it overhead by extending your arms.
- Holding the ViPR overhead, with arms extended and your abdominals braced, step backwards with your right leg into the reverse lunge position.
- Maintain correct tension in your core muscles and shoulders to keep the ViPR stable as you lower into the lunge.
- Before your right knee reaches the floor behind you, pause briefly before pushing back up using your glutes and quads to return to a standing position with feet hip-distance apart.

- Lower the ViPR carefully to your chest and then to the waist.
- Finally, lower to touch the floor without letting go before bracing your abdominals again and repeating the clean and press action, to hold the ViPR above your head before lunging back, this time with your left leg.
- Repeat the complete movement, alternating between left and right legs for a total of 10–20 repetitions.

Modifications

- Perform the clean and press action from a 'hang clean' position, with the ViPR held at waist height instead of touching the floor.
- Repeat the clean and press action with the reverse lunges before lowering to waist height and repeating.

Ex 10.32 ViPR uppercut lunges

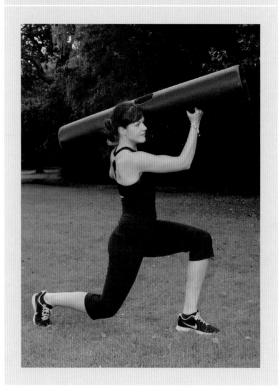

- Repeat, this time stepping forwards into a lunge position with your right leg, pushing the ViPR so that your right hand is over your left in an 'uppercut' movement leading with your left arm.
- Return to the start position, pushing back off your right leg.
- Repeat 10–15 times each side.

Starting position and action
- Hold the ViPR by the grips, in front of your chest, with your arms bent and abdominals braced.
- Initially, rotate the ViPR 90 degrees into a vertical position with your left hand above your right hand.
- Simultaneously step forward with your left leg into a lunge position as you push your right hand forwards, holding the ViPR in an 'upper-cut' action.
- Slow the ViPR movement and pull back with your right hand, maintaining core tension as you push back off your left leg from the lunge to return back to the starting position.

Ex 10.33 ViPR uppercuts to block

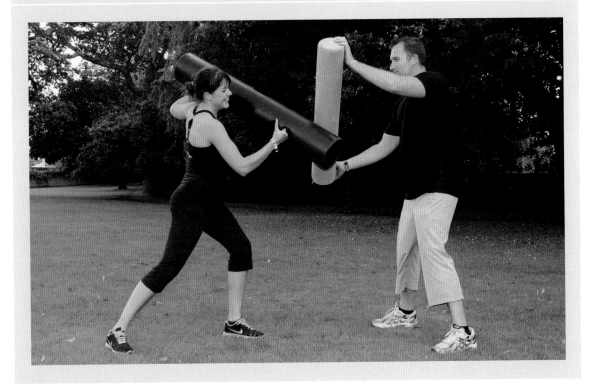

Starting position and action

- This drill really applies the dynamics of power when using a ViPR.
- Begin holding the ViPR with both hands in front of your chest, with your abdominals braced and your elbows slightly bent, as in the uppercut lunge. Your partner should hold his own ViPR and face you.
- Step forwards with your right leg into a partial-lunge position as you rotate the ViPR through 90 degrees and continue this movement, pushing the ViPR upwards with your left arm in a forceful 'uppercut' movement to contact your partner's ViPR.

- Push back off your front leg and pull back with your left arm to rotate the ViPR back to the start position.
- Then repeat the movement, stepping forwards with your left leg rotating the ViPR and push it with your right arm in an uppercut movement to forcefully contact your partner's ViPR.
- Do alternate partial lunges and uppercuts 12–20 times each side.

Modifications

- You can vary the direction of 'strike' and force applied in the uppercuts together with the degree of torso rotation while performing the uppercut movement.

Ex **10.34** ViPR body pulls

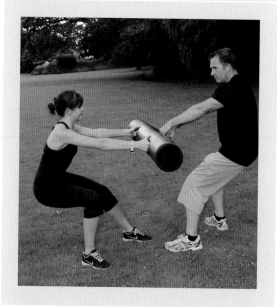

Ex **10.35** ViPR body pushes

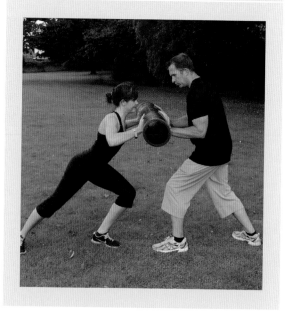

Starting position and action

- Stand holding on to the grips of a ViPR held at chest height with arms outstretched, feet in a split-stance and knees slightly bent.
- Lean back to take the strain of the ViPR being held by your partner and begin to pull backwards, pushing off with your legs and pulling with your arms.
- Keep your abdominals braced throughout and maintain an upright posture as you aim to drag your partner, pushing off from your legs and pulling with your arms.
- Aim to drag the ViPR and your partner over a distance of 10–15m before resting and repeating.
- It is important that your partner works with you and allows you to be sufficiently challenged yet able to complete the exercise over the desired distance in 20–30 seconds before recovering and repeating for another 3–5 attempts.

Starting position and action

- Stand as before, holding on to the grips of a ViPR held at chest height, this time with arms bent and elbows behind it, ready to push.
- Keep your feet in a split-stance, knees slightly bent, and lean forwards to begin to push against your partner.
- Your partner places their hands on the ViPR and resists you.
- Keep your abdominals braced throughout and do not hold your breath as you push.
- As in the previous exercise, your partner needs to work with you to provide adequate resistance to push against but still allow you to perform the movement across the area in 20–30 seconds before recovering and repeating a further 3–5 attempts.

Ex 10.36 ViPR longitudinal drags

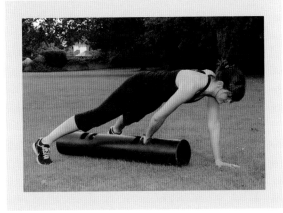

Ex 10.37 ViPR horizontal drags

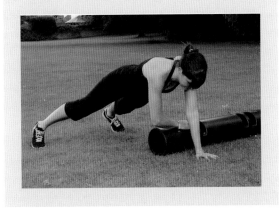

Starting position and action

- Position yourself in a prone position, your bodyweight supported through your arms and legs.
- With the ViPR under your torso, brace your abdominals and take hold of it with your right hand.
- Pull the ViPR forwards to drag it towards your chest using your right hand, while remaining in the prone position.
- Once you have dragged the ViPR forwards, walk forwards on your hands and feet, still in the prone position, about 0.5m with the ViPR still underneath you.
- This time drag the ViPR forwards, keeping your abdominals braced, using your left hand.
- Repeat the 'drag and walk forwards' technique 10–15 times or over a distance of 15–20m.

Starting position and action

- Position yourself prone on your hands with arms extended and with legs outstretched behind you as before.
- The ViPR should be perpendicular to your torso, underneath your chest but close enough so that you can reach the grips.
- With feet and hands shoulder-width apart, lift your right arm, taking your weight on to your left arm and legs, and hold the grips of the ViPR with your right hand.
- Keeping your abdominals braced, drag the ViPR from underneath you to the right about 1m.
- Then place your right hand back on the floor and reach underneath yourself with your left hand to grab the ViPR, and then drag the ViPR approximately to your left.
- Repeat right and left 'drags' 15–20 times.

Ex 10.38 ViPR 'thread the needle'

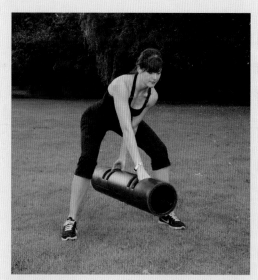

Modification

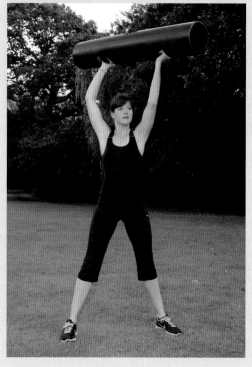

Starting position and action

- Hold the ViPR at arms' length with it resting on your thighs.
- Bracing your abdominals, lift the ViPR to chest height as you squat down and rotate the ViPR 90 degrees, to 'feed' it between your legs, leading with your right hand.
- Slow the ViPR movement down and reverse the action, maintaining abdominal tension, and then drive the ViPR back up to chest height, rotating the ViPR anti-clockwise at chest height with arms outstretched in front of you.
- Repeat movement by squatting down again, to thread the ViPR between your legs, this time leading with the left hand. Maintain abdominal bracing throughout.
- Repeat movement for 10–20 complete reps.

Modifications

- To progress the exercise, you can lift the ViPR overhead to rotate 180 degrees before squatting down to repeat the entire movement.
- To progress further, change your footprint by adding a quarter turn or half turn when the ViPR is above your head or even jump into a quarter-turn or half-turn position, thus rotating 90 or 180 degrees before repeating the movement sequence.

Ex 10.39 ViPR canoe/kayak rows

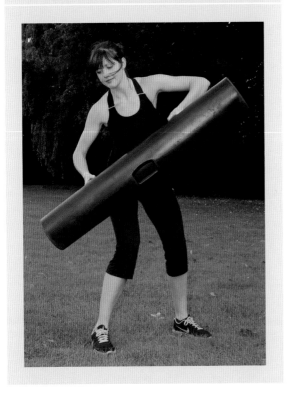

- Complete 20–30 alternating figure-8 movements before placing the ViPR on the floor to finish.

Modifications
- This exercise can be performed in a standing or seated position, either on a bench, stability ball, BOSU, or seated on the floor with your knees bent.
- Increase the intensity by using a heavier ViPR or by simply increasing the speed of 'paddling'.

Starting position and action
- In this exercise, the ViPR follows a similar movement to that of a paddle being held by a canoeist or kayaker, yet the resistance of the ViPR obviously makes the entire movement far more demanding.
- Stand with your feet hip-distance apart, hold the ViPR in front of you with your arms bent.
- With your abdominals braced, rotate the ViPR in a figure-8 movement, as if paddling a canoe, with each end of the ViPR performing small circles to either side as you rotate it.
- Ensure that you maintain correct abdominal bracing throughout without holding your breath.

Ex 10.40 ViPR squat and sweeps

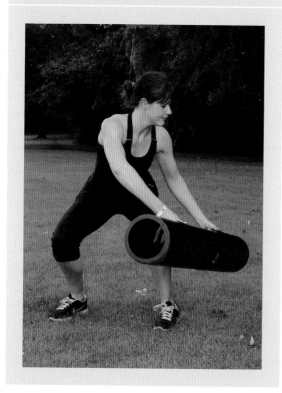

Starting position and action

- Hold a ViPR horizontally with your arms bent at 90 degrees, feet shoulder-width apart and your abdominals braced.
- Slowly squat down, by bending your knees and sitting back while simultaneously rotating and moving the ViPR to your left side in a 'sweeping' movement, not dissimilar to a paddling action.
- Pause briefly in the squat position with your thighs almost parallel to the floor and the ViPR held outside your left hip, with your torso partially rotated to your left and arms still bent.

- Then straighten your legs to return to a standing position, bringing the ViPR back to the start position, ensuring your abdominals are braced throughout.
- From the standing position, this time squat down and rotate the ViPR to your right side, twisting at the waist to your right.
- In the squat position, pause briefly and then return to standing, bringing the ViPR back to the start position with your arms bent at 90 degrees.

Modifications

- This exercise can be intensified by increasing the speed of movement and increasing the rotation aspect to push the ViPR further to your side and slightly behind you, extending your arms slightly as you do so.

Ex 10.41 ViPR ice skater

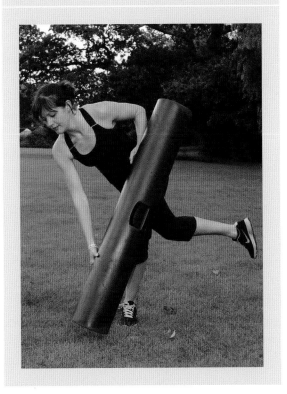

- Repeat alternate lateral stepping movements with the ViPR rotations for 12–20 repetitions each side.

Modifications

- To increase the intensity, increase the speed of side-stepping and pressing the ViPR to each side, building up from side-steps to dynamic leaps to each side, hopping right and left with greater distance.

Starting position and action

- Hold the ViPR at arms' length in front of you with your feet shoulder-width apart and your knees slightly bent.
- Keeping your abdominals braced throughout, step with your left leg laterally to your left.
- As you step, rotate the ViPR, pushing down with your right hand to change the ViPR's position from horizontal to almost vertical, with your left hand over your right.
- As you step, decelerate the movement of the ViPR before reversing the action, rotating in the other direction as you step laterally to your right.

Ex 10.42 ViPR overhead squats with tilt

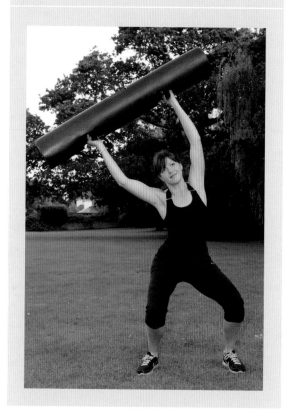

left, pausing briefly, returning to the overhead position and standing up.
- Repeat the squat and tilt movement for a total of 10–20 repetitions.

Modifications
- To reduce the intensity you could tilt the ViPR when standing upright as opposed to during the squat.
- Another option is to perform the full clean-and-press action before each squat and tilt, making this a very demanding total-body exercise.

Starting position and action
- Begin holding the ViPR above your head with your arms extended and squat down to a near-seated position, with your thighs almost parallel to the floor, with the ViPR held overhead.
- Pause briefly and then tilt the ViPR to your right to change the centre of balance and stabilisation required through your core muscles.
- Return the ViPR to an overhead position before returning to a standing position, keeping the ViPR over your head throughout.
- Repeat the squat but this time, when in the lowered squat position, tilt the ViPR to the

Ex 10.43 ViPR multi-direction lunges

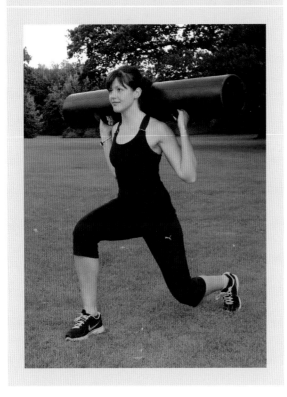

Starting position and action
- Begin standing with feet shoulder-width apart and holding a ViPR across your shoulders.
- Take a lunge and step diagonally forwards with your right leg, maintaining abdominal tension throughout.
- As your right leg touches the floor, bend both knees and lunge down until your right thigh is almost parallel to the floor, keeping your torso upright and holding the ViPR horizontal across your shoulders.
- Pause briefly at the lower part of the lunge and then return back to the start position.

- Repeat, this time with your left leg lunging diagonally out to your left, changing the angle of the lunge.
- Repeat alternate lunges, varying the direction of lunge to either side, making sure you keep your torso upright with abdominals braced.

Modifications
- In addition to forward and diagonal lunges, you can perform reverse and reverse-diagonal lunges, stepping back with both right and left legs.
- To increase the stabilisation and intensity when in the lunge position, perform an overhead press with the ViPR while maintaining correct tension throughout the torso.
- To add greater stabilisation to the movement, when you push back to the start position add a knee lift with the moving leg so that you are balancing on one leg while keeping your abdominals braced and the ViPR on your shoulders or held overhead.

KETTLEBELL DRILLS

Kettlebells are essentially big cannonball-shaped weights with handles and have been used in strength conditioning for over 100 years. While most classic dumbbell exercises can be performed using a kettlebell, they really come into their own with forceful dynamic movements such as swings, cleans and snatches and combinations of all of these. The nature of these movements require the core muscles, shoulders and *lumbo-pelvic hip complex* to work in unison and, as such, many kettlebell exercises are excellent total-body exercises that challenge not only your muscles but your cardiovascular system as well, due to the nature of the repeated lifts and swings with the heavy resistance. The kettlebell swing action is an excellent posterior chain exercise, in that it works all the muscles of the lower back, hamstrings and calves.

Ex 10.44 Kettlebell swings

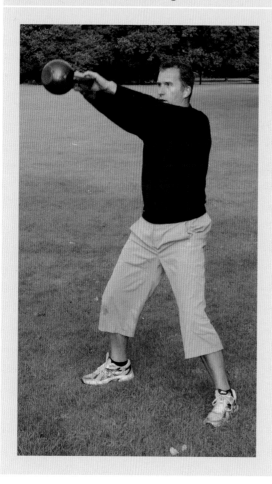

Starting position and action

- Pick up the kettlebell with both hands on the handle, maintaining tension through your core muscles to protect your back as you lift.
- Holding the kettlebell at waist height with arms straight, retract your shoulders to counter the weight of the bell.
- Thrust your hips forwards to push the kettlebell away from the body, propelling it forward, and then lower it, swinging it through your knees with knees bent, flexing your hips and leaning forward slightly with your backside pushed backwards.
- Then drive your hips forwards, ensuring your abdominals are braced throughout, and contract your glutes to propel the kettlebell upwards to approximately chest height as you return back to a standing position.
- Repeat the 'swinging' action 15–25 times, before lowering the kettlebell to the floor.
- Remember to keep breathing throughout the swinging action, exhaling as you apply the force through your hips and glutes to propel it upwards.

Ex 10.45 Single-arm swings

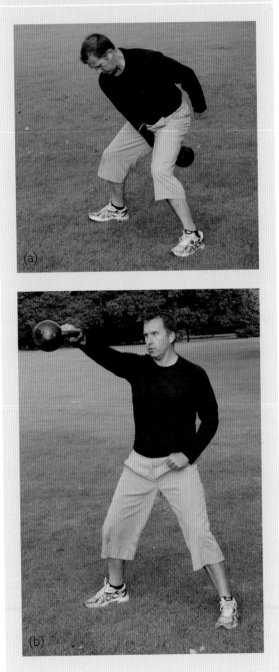

(a)

(b)

Starting position and action

- Follow the same movements as in Ex 10.44, yet hold the kettlebell in your right hand only and perform 10–15 swings before changing to your left hand and repeating for another 10–15 swings.
- For the single-arm swings, when you swing the kettlebell between your legs rotate the kettlebell 90 degrees inwards by pronating your forearm so that your thumb points downwards and towards you.
- Your 'free' arm is generally used for balance during all the swinging actions, and can be held at various positions – in front of you, placed in the small of your lower back or even above your head, which places different stabilisation demands on your core muscles.

Ex 10.46 Alternating single-arm swings

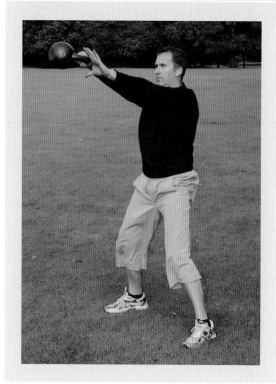

Ex 10.47 Single-arm kettlebell clean and racks

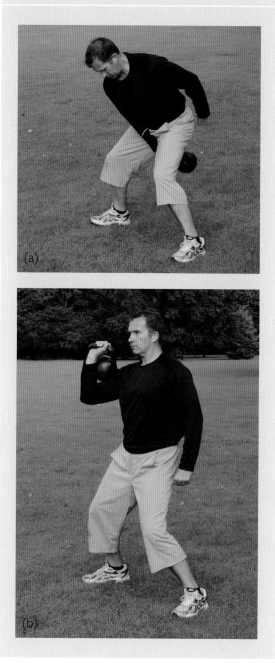

(a)

(b)

Starting position and action

- This technique is a variation to the single-arm swing, whereby at the top point of the movement, where the kettlebell has been swung to approximately chest height, you change hands quickly from right to left before rotating the kettlebell inwards and lowering to swing back between your legs.
- Repeat this action 20–30 times.

Starting position and action

- Stand over the kettlebell with your feet shoulder-width apart.
- Reach down with one hand to take hold of the kettlebell, keeping your abdominals braced.
- Swing the kettlebell between your legs, with your thumb inwards, before forcefully thrusting your hips forwards to powerfully drive the kettlebell upwards in an arc movement.
- When the kettlebell reaches slightly above shoulder height, bend your legs to lower your body as you drop your elbow and 'flip' your wrist underneath the kettlebell.
- The kettlebell should 'land' midway between your elbow and shoulder on your upper arm, with your elbow tucked in.
- This end position is called the 'rack' position and is the start position for all pressing movement overhead.
- From this 'rack' position, pause briefly before rotating the kettlebell and lowering down in a swinging action back to the start position.
- Repeat for 10–15 complete 'clean and rack' moves before changing hands and repeating.
- When in the rack position, ensure the kettlebell handle is held in the palm of your hand, next to your thumb, in preparation for pressing movements with which you can follow.

Ex 10.48 Single-arm clean and presses

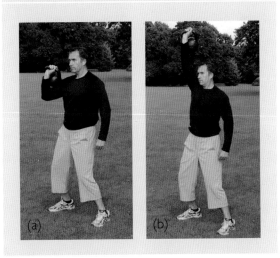

(a)   (b)

Starting position and action

- Take hold of the kettlebell in one hand as before, bracing your abdominals before swinging and dropping down to flip the kettlebell into the 'rack' position on your upper arm in preparation to press.
- In this position, standing upright and with your abdominals braced, extend your arm to push the kettlebell overhead, keeping your forearm vertical and elbow facing forward.
- Once the kettlebell is overhead, lower it back to the 'rack' position, before rotating it and lowering it down in a swinging action as before.
- Repeat the clean, rack and press action 10–15 times before lowering the kettlebell and repeating with your opposite hand.
- Ensure you keep your core muscles activated throughout and maintain regular breathing without holding your breath.

Ex 10.49 Single-arm snatch and squats

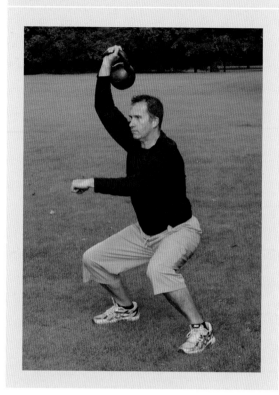

- As the kettlebell reaches shoulder height, 'sink' slightly by bending your knees, and 'punch' through the kettlebell, to continue the upward swing so that you finish with your right arm locked and the kettlebell held overhead.
- With the kettlebell now above your head and arm extended, squat down, keeping your back in neutral alignment, with your abdominals braced.
- From the squat position, with abdominals braced, push through your heels to return to a standing position, with your arm still extended and the kettlebell over your head.
- Then carefully lower the kettlebell, rolling on to your forearm into the rack position before lowering back to the floor. Repeat the 'snatch and squat' technique 10–15 times.
- Repeat with your left hand for another 10–15 complete repetitions.

Starting position and action
- Stand over the kettlebell with your feet shoulder-width apart and bend down, bracing your abdominals to lift the kettlebell, driving up through your legs and hips to push the kettlebell outwards.
- When it swings back through your legs, maintain core tension and correct alignment as you lean forwards, bending your legs before forcefully thrusting your hips forwards to swing the kettlebell upwards in an arc.

Ex 10.50 Overhead lunges

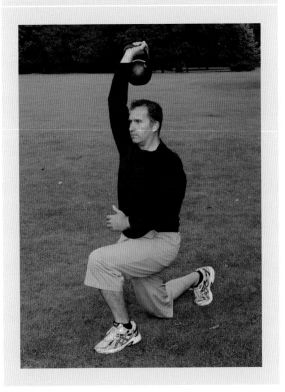

Repeat the clean, rack and press sequence to hold the kettlebell overhead in your left hand and repeat the reverse lunge movement, stepping back with your left leg, before pushing back up using your right thigh and glutes to return to standing. Perform another 10–15 repetitions before lowering the kettlebell to the floor.

Starting position and action

- Perform the clean, rack and press technique to lift the kettlebell above your head in the standing position.
- Holding the kettlebell with your arm extended overhead, lunge backwards with your right leg to lower towards the ground, keeping your weight over your front leg.
- Then push through your glutes and thigh, returning yourself back to a standing position.
- Repeat 10–15 times before lowering the kettlebell and changing hands.

Ex 10.51 Kettlebell Turkish get-ups

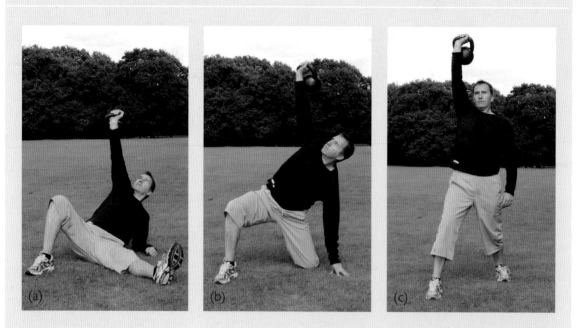

(a)   (b)   (c)

Starting position and action

- This is a very demanding exercise and requires balance, strength and fitness to keep repeating the movement. It will strengthen your hips, glutes, legs and shoulders.
- Lie on your back holding a kettlebell in your right hand above your chest, with your elbow locked.
- Bend your right knee to bring your right foot towards your glutes, knee bent at 90 degrees.
- With your left arm out to the side and your hand on the floor, push the kettlebell into the air, keeping your abdominals braced and push your right foot into the floor as you lift your chest, leaning on your supporting left forearm.
- Push your right heel into the floor and lift up your hips to allow you to pull your left leg underneath and behind you to bring you into a

kneeling position on your left knee. Hold the kettlebell overhead throughout.
- When you are balanced, take your left hand off the floor, maintaining your core tension as you hold the kneeling lunge position.
- While still holding the kettlebell above your head, push up through your glutes and quads to stand up using your free arm to assist your balance.
- From standing, repeat the entire process in reverse, ensuring you are bracing the abdominals throughout to return back down to the floor.
- Aim for 5–8 repetitions before swapping the kettlebell to your opposite hand and repeating again from the floor position.

Ex **10.52** Kettlebell halos

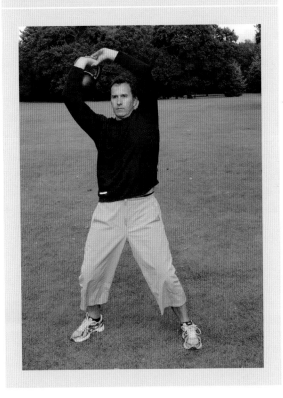

your head and then lower back to the left and then swing back right.

- Continue these full movements and swings for 6–10 complete rotations to each side then squat down and lower the kettlebell under control to the floor.

Modifications

- Focus on just the rotation part of the movement by 'rotating' the kettlebell clockwise around your head for 8–12 repetitions before slowing the movement and then reversing the direction to rotate the kettlebell 8–12 rotations in an anti-clockwise direction.
- After completing these rotations, lower the kettlebell down to the floor under control, maintaining correct core tension throughout.
- An alternative is to lift the kettlebell from the floor each time, so that you squat down and lift the kettlebell then rotate it around your head before lowering back to the floor, before lifting again and rotating it in the opposite direction.

Starting position and action

- Bend down and grasp the kettlebell. Keeping your back fairly straight, push through your legs and glutes to a standing position, keeping your abdominals braced.
- With your legs slightly bent and abdominals braced, swing the kettlebell to the left side and as it swings back down and to the right, bend your arms to lift and rotate the kettlebell around your head once before lowering it back down and to the right side and then left.
- Then, maintaining this bottom phase swing, swing the kettlebell initially to the right and then as it swings back to the left, bend your arms and rotate the kettlebell back around

Ex 10.53 Kettlebell clean and racks on BOSU

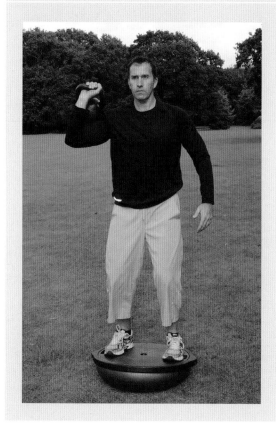

land midway between your elbow and shoulder on your upper right arm and with your elbow tucked in.

- Pause briefly in the 'rack' position before rotating the kettlebell and lowering down in a swinging action, again leading through your legs, thumb first.
- Repeat the complete action 10–20 times before changing grip and repeating holding the kettlebell in your left hand.
- On completion, lower the kettlebell to waist height and then step off the BOSU and lower the kettlebell to the floor.

Starting position and action

- Begin standing on the BOSU (flat side up) holding a kettlebell in your right hand, with your feet shoulder-width apart.
- Brace your abdominals and swing the kettlebell between your legs, with your thumb pointing inwards before extending through your hips and legs to powerfully drive the kettlebell upwards, lifting it in an arc movement.
- Then 'sink' slightly by bending your legs as you drop your right elbow and 'flip' your wrist underneath the kettlebell to rotate it over to

Ex 10.54 Kettlebell push-ups with row

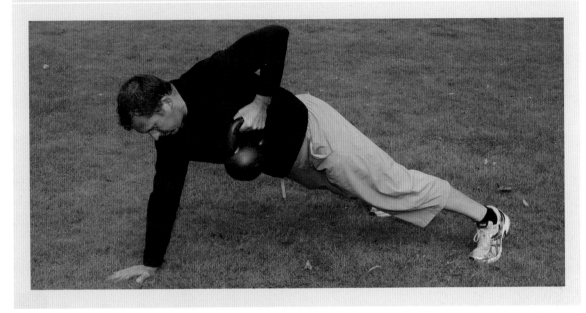

Starting position and action

- Position yourself in a prone position with legs outstretched behind you and your arms shoulder-width apart, so that your weight is supported through your right hand on the floor and your left hand holding the kettlebell.
- Maintain abdominal bracing, keeping your torso in a fixed position with spine in neutral alignment.
- Slowly bend both your arms, ensuring you maintain rigidity through your torso and keeping the kettlebell handle upright, which is supporting your bodyweight.
- Lower your chest towards the ground and then extend your arms, pushing through your chest, shoulders and triceps to return back to the start position.
- In this position, keeping your abdominals braced, take your weight on to your right arm and lift the kettlebell in your left hand towards your ribcage.
- Pause briefly, holding the kettlebell next to your chest and rotating your body slightly to your right to assist balance.
- Then lower the kettlebell back to the floor underneath your left shoulder.
- Perform push-up rows 15–20 times before repeating with the kettlebell in your right hand.

Modifications

- Another option is to perform the push-up row using two kettlebells, doing a push-up while holding both handles and then lifting the kettlebells alternately to you ribs after each push-up.
- To reduce the stabilisation requirement, use dumbbells instead of kettlebells.
- To reduce the intensity of the press-up, perform it on your knees.

Ex 10.55 Single-arm balance rows

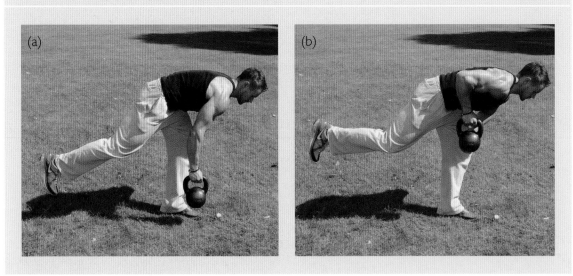

Starting position and action

- Stand holding a kettlebell in your right hand, keeping your abdominals braced.
- Bend your left leg slightly and lean forwards at the waist to lower your torso to almost a horizontal position, while holding the kettlebell with your right arm hanging down.
- Keeping correct bracing throughout your torso, with your right leg in the air behind you, contract your biceps muscles and upper back muscles to pull the kettlebell towards your chest.
- Pause briefly with the kettlebell handle touching your ribs and then lower back to the start position.
- Repeat 12–20 times before changing hands.
- Repeat exercise with the kettlebell in your left hand, but bend your right leg and lean forwards as before. This time your left leg will be behind you in the air.

- Pull the kettlebell to your chest as before 12–20 times before returning to standing position and then bend your legs and place the kettlebell on the floor in front of you.

SUSPENSION TRAINING® DRILLS

Suspension straps are fantastic when used in an outdoor environment, as they are light and portable. They are suitable for all fitness levels and by simple adjustments of your stance and body position, you can intensify or reduce the intensity of every exercise.

They were originally the brain child of a US Navy Seal who created prototypes based on parachutes. Consequently, the device consists of nylon straps, grips and a carabiner to secure the locking mechanism. You wrap the nylon straps or cables over a solid object such as a lamppost, high bar, tree or anything that is secure, and that will then take your bodyweight as you lean away from the anchor point. You have to maintain a relatively rigid torso and so they are a fantastic aid to training your core stability. This *total-body integration* of muscles helps enhance joint stability, muscular balance and improved mobility.

Ex 10.56 Suspended atomic push-ups

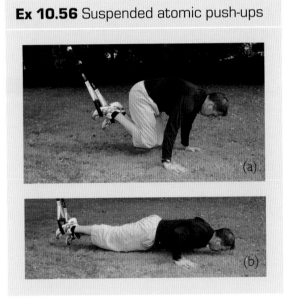

(a)

(b)

arms and shoulders into a suspended crunch position.
- Then extend your legs back behind you and perform a push-up, lowering your chest to the floor by bending your arms.
- When your chest is about 15cm from the floor, push yourself back to the start position, maintaining correct spinal alignment.
- Repeat the knees-to-chest action with full press-up for 10–20 complete movements.

Modifications
- Perform an oblique crunch instead of a suspended crunch, followed by the full push-up in outstretched position.
- For the oblique crunch, twist your torso slightly and draw your knees in, but to your right side, before returning back to the straight leg position and performing a push-up.
- Next time draw your knees in to your left side before extending your legs and performing the push-up.
- Repeat this alternating oblique crunch with full push-ups for a total of 8–15 complete movements to each side.

Starting position and action
- Place your feet in the suspension cradles and rotate over to your right side to position yourself on your hands, placed slightly wider than shoulder-width apart.
- Keeping your abdominals braced, draw your knees in towards your chest, lifting your hips and supporting your bodyweight through your

Ex 10.57 Suspended single-arm power pulls with rotation

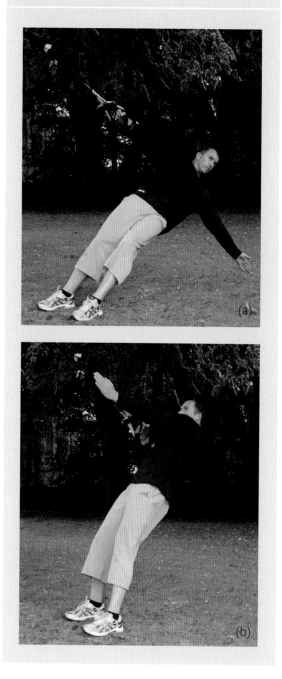

(a)

(b)

Starting position and action

- Secure the handles by interlocking them, and hold one handle with your right hand in front of you.
- Lean back, holding the handle with your arm fully extended, and rotate to your left so that you can reach down with your left hand towards the floor.
- Pull yourself up towards the handle using your upper back muscles and arm, keeping your abdominals braced and torso rigid throughout.
- As you pull yourself towards the handle, turn your torso inwards, reaching over and across with your left hand to reach towards the anchor point, holding this position briefly before returning back to the start position.
- Repeat 10–20 times before changing hands and doing the exercise with your left hand.

Ex 10.58 Suspended total body burpees

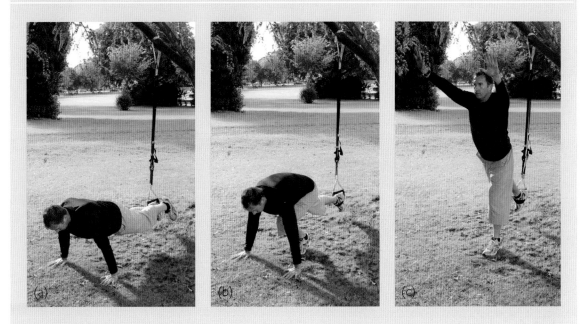

(a)   (b)   (c)

Starting position and action

- Interlock the handles to create a fixed handle and from a seated position, feed your right foot through the foot cradle. Turn over to place your hands on the floor, slightly wider than shoulder-width apart, with your right foot suspended in the cable.
- Brace your abdominals and lift your left leg off the floor to bring it adjacent to your right, ensuring your hips are stabilised.
- Perform a push-up, lowering your chest to the floor by bending your elbows and then extending your arms.
- Then bring your left knee back in towards your chest and placing your left foot on the floor, under your hips.
- Push up with your left leg and arms into a standing position.
- Repeat the complete movement as before, lowering back to the ground, extending your left leg and performing another push-up.
- Repeat for 8–15 repetitions before changing your suspended leg and repeating, this time with your left leg in the cradle, maintaining correct form throughout.

191

Ex 10.59 Stabilisation hangs

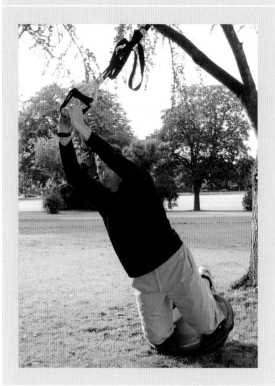

Pause briefly before returning across to lean to your right side.

• Repeat alternate leans 20–30 times.

Modifications
• This exercise can be enhanced by leaning at different angles, not just left and right but also at a 45-degree angle forwards and backwards, and even taking this to a 360-degree option whereby you lean at any angle, providing you can control the movement and maintain abdominal tension throughout.
• If the BOSU proves too much of a challenge, try while kneeling on the ground.

Starting position and action
• Firstly, loop the handles of a cable through one another to create a secured single-handle grip.
• Kneel on a BOSU (flat side up) while holding on to this single handle with both hands clasped together over your head, arms outstretched.
• While holding the handle, keeping your abdominals braced, lean across to your right side to allow more of your bodyweight to be taken through your arms.
• Hold this unstable position briefly before tilting back across to your left side, still holding on to the handle with arms overhead.

Ex **10.60** Suspended T-deltoid raises

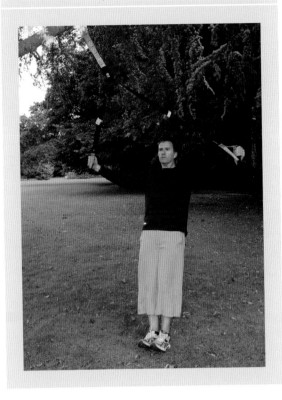

Starting position and action

- Hold the grips at arms' length, facing the anchor point, and lean back so that your bodyweight is supported, while maintaining core stability through your torso muscles and shoulder complex.
- With your feet together, pull on the grips by separating your arms out perpendicular to your torso to lift your body upwards toward the anchor point.
- Keep your body rigid throughout the movement.
- Repeat for 12–20 complete movements.

Ex **10.61** Suspended Y-deltoid raises

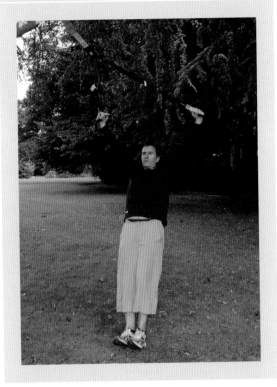

Starting position and action

- A variation to the 'T' position described in exercise 10.60 is the Y-deltoid raise which, as the name implies, takes your arms into a 'Y' position.
- This places more emphasis on your shoulders and so your initial start position might need adjusting.
- Begin as before, facing the anchor point and holding the straps, yet this time pull your arms up and outwards at a diagonal to your torso to lift your body towards the anchor point, keeping your body rigid throughout.

Ex 10.62 Suspended single-leg squats

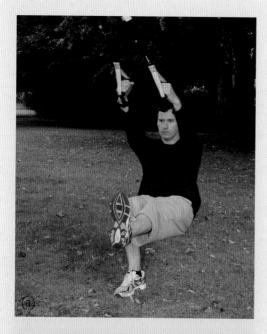

(a)

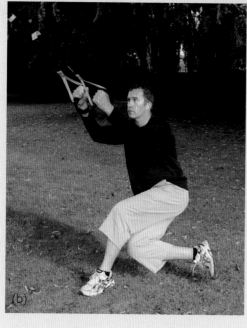

(b)

Starting position and action

- Hold the handles with both arms extended, leaning back facing the anchor point, with your feet hip-distance apart.
- Keeping your abdominals braced, lift your left leg off the floor to transfer your bodyweight on to your right leg.
- Sit back, bending your right leg to lower yourself into a single-leg squatting position, holding the handles.
- Repeat 12–20 times before changing your supporting leg and repeating on your left leg.

Modification: Dynamic lunge

- A more dynamic movement is to jump alternately to your right and then left foot, performing the single-leg squat, but forcefully pushing up and off your leg to land on your other leg and repeating the single-leg squat.
- Aim for power and height with each push, repeating 15–30 times.
- Increase this by adding distance and lateral movement to each jump.

Modification: Balanced lunge

- The balance lunge is a variation of the dynamic single-leg squats where your 'free' leg goes behind and to the outside of your supporting leg as you squat down (Ex 10.62b).
- Be careful not to lose abdominal bracing as you perform this movement.
- The movement of your raised leg will affect your hip and pelvis alignment, so try not to extend your raised leg too far behind your squatting leg.

Ex **10.63** Suspended dips

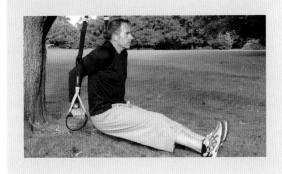

Ex **10.64** Suspended hip presses

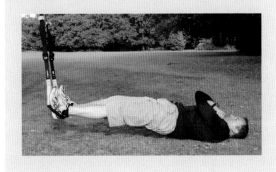

Starting position and action

- Hold on to the grips of the cables with your feet outstretched in front of you in a modified seated position, with your bodyweight supported through your arms and shoulders, holding the grips in your hands, legs slightly bent.
- Stabilise your shoulders and arms to stop the straps from moving and then slowly bend your elbows to lower into a triceps dip.
- If you can, lower to a 90-degree flexion at the elbow, while maintaining control and then push back up, contracting your triceps to lift you back to the start position.
- Repeat 10–20 times.

Modifications

- To reduce the intensity, position the handles further from the floor by shortening the straps, so that more of your bodyweight is supported through your legs.
- To intensify this drill, place your feet on a raised platform, such as a bench, or to increase intensity and the stabilisation challenge, place your feet on a medicine ball or BOSU.

Starting position and action

- From a seated position, place your heels into the straps with the cradle about 20–25cm from the floor.
- Lie back on to the ground and extend your legs, with your arms by your side.
- Bracing your abdominals, lift your backside off the floor, pushing your hips upwards.
- Hold briefly in the top position before lowering back to the ground, before repeating again.
- Repeat hip-press action 10–20 times before resting.
- To assist in stabilising, keep your arms on the floor and as you progress, cross your arms over your chest.

TRX® RIP™ TRAINER DRILLS

The Rip Trainer utilises a lever bar attached at one end to a variable resistance cord, which is secured to an anchor point to create resistance when the cord is stretched. It allows almost unlimited movement opportunities, incorporating lower-body movements, such as squats, lunges, stepping and jumping movements, together with upper-body movements, such as pulling, pressing, throwing and rotational movements. The combined outcome of these multi-planar dynamic movements is to train not only your core muscles, but to integrate all muscles within the movement to improve your strength, power, co-ordination and balance.

The main difference of the TRX® Rip™ Trainer compared to other equipment is that it is asymmetrically loaded so that the applied force is on one end, which consequently requires you to stabilise the other end, leading to greater total-muscle integration.

If you perform dynamic exercises with the Rip Trainer, it can help to train your power, co-ordination and motor skill (use the lower resistance cord), whereas if you perform slower exercises with greater control at a reduced speed (use the higher resistance cord) you challenge your strength and core stability.

In a similar manner to the ViPR, you can combine the TRX® Rip™ Trainer with unstable bases, such as a BOSU, to create movements that enhance fluidity and range of motion, which really challenge your stabilising muscles and balance.

Ex 10.65 TRX® Rip™ Trainer squats to high row

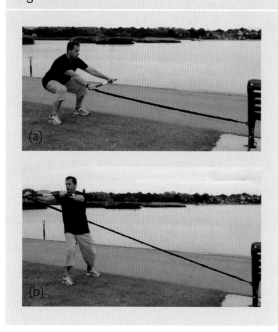

Starting position and action

- Hold on to the lever bar at arms' length facing the anchor point, with your feet hip-distance apart and the resistance cord to your right.
- Brace your abdominals and slowly squat down, trying not to lean forwards.
- Then as you stand back up, keep your abdominals braced, pull on the bar, rotating to your right, and lift the lever bar to approximately shoulder height.
- Return to the start position and squat down as before.
- Repeat these squats and high rows, rotating to your right each time for 15–20 repetitions, before changing grips and holding the lever bar with the resistance cord attached to the left side.
- Repeat squat and high rows again, this time rotating to your left side 15–20 times.

Ex 10.66 TRX® Rip™ Trainer squats to low row

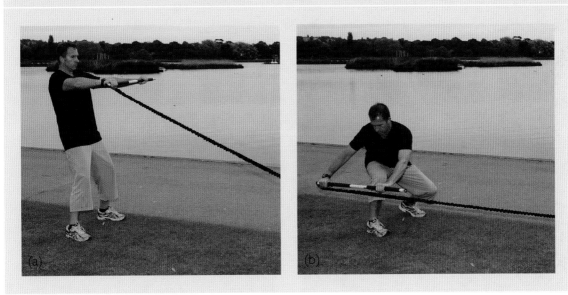
(a) (b)

Starting position and action

- The squat and low row is similar to the previous exercise, yet the row movement is performed during the squat action.
- Stand as before, facing the anchor point and holding the lever bar, with the resistance cord to your right.
- Brace your abdominals and sit back to squat down. As you reach the lower position, pull on the lever bar and rotate to your right side.
- Slowly rotate the bar back and stand up, returning to the start position.
- Repeat the squat and row technique 15–20 times before changing your grip so that the resistance cord is on the left and repeat for another 15–20 repetitions, this time squatting and rotating to your left.

Ex 10.67 TRX® Rip™ Trainer squats to asymmetric press

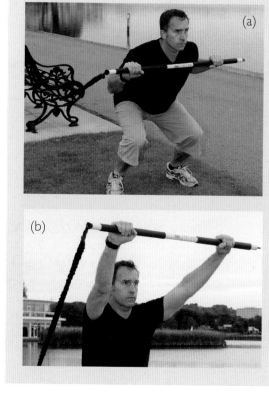

(a)

(b)

Starting position and action

- Hold on to the lever bar with the resistance tube secured behind you.
- Stand in a neutral stance, holding the lever bar with the resistance tube to your right.
- Bracing your abdominals, lift the bar to shoulder height in front of your chest and squat down until your thighs are almost parallel to the floor, pausing briefly at the lowered position, keeping your spine in neutral alignment.
- Then dynamically push back up to a standing position, pressing the TRX® Rip™ Trainer bar upwards and slightly forwards, keeping your arms in alignment with your body to press the bar overhead.
- Lower the lever bar back to shoulder height and squat back down as before.
- Repeat the squat and press action 10–15 times with the TRX® Rip™ Trainer attached to the right of the bar, before resting and then repeating for another 15–20 repetitions, this time with the resistance to your left side.
- The asymmetric nature of pull on this exercise means your abdominals will be challenged laterally and you will need to maintain correct core tension throughout to keep correct posture and alignment.

Modifications

- Try varying your stance for this exercise and performing the squat action with feet in a split-stance or staggered-stance position, one foot in front of the other.
- Alternatively, perform the squat with feet hip-distance or closer apart.
- To challenge your stabilisation even further, perform the squat on a BOSU.
- This exercise can involve rotation by standing sideways on to the anchor point and holding the lever bar to your chest. After performing a squat, rotate and step forwards with your right leg to face away from the anchor point as you press the lever bar forwards and above your head. Then step back and rotate back to the start position before squatting down again and repeating.
- To add a greater dynamic, with or without the rotation element, you could jump into the position as you press the lever bar above your head, adding increased resistance forces and stabilisation requirements.

Ex 10.68 TRX® Rip™ Trainer lunges to stand with shoulder press

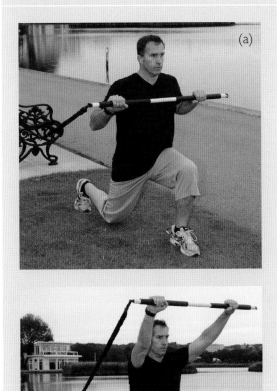

(a)

(b)

Starting position and action

- Anchor the base of the TRX® Rip™ Trainer and stand facing away from the anchor point, holding the lever bar with both hands at chest height, approximately shoulder-width apart.
- Your feet should be slightly staggered with toes pointing forwards.

- Holding the bar to your chest, with abdominals braced, step back into a reverse lunge with your right leg, bending both knees to lower your body towards the floor.
- As your left thigh reaches a horizontal position and before your right knee touches the floor, keeping your abdominals braced, push through your left leg and buttocks to return to a standing position while extending your arms to press the lever bar upwards at a 45–60 degree angle, away from the anchor point.
- As you step up from the lunge position, bring your right leg parallel to your left leg.
- Then lower the bar back towards your chest and shoulders while stepping back, this time with your left leg into a reverse lunge position.
- At the lower position, extend through your right leg and hips to return to a standing position, bringing your left leg back to parallel with your right.
- At the same time extend your arms, pushing the bar upwards as before, working your arms, shoulders and chest but maintaining abdominal bracing throughout.
- Repeat alternate lunges and presses for 15–20 repetitions.

Modifications

- Perform the reverse lunge on the same leg for 8–12 repetitions before changing legs and repeating on the other leg.
- Because the TRX® Rip™ Trainer is attached on one side, you can vary lunging and pressing with either leg with the resistance cable on your right side and then the lever bar across to the other side so that the 'pull' is from the other side.

Ex 10.69 TRX® Rip™ Trainer axe chops

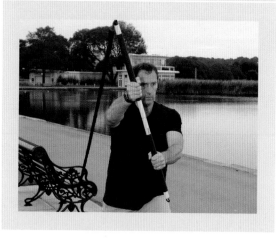

Ex 10.70 TRX® Rip™ Trainer seated chest presses

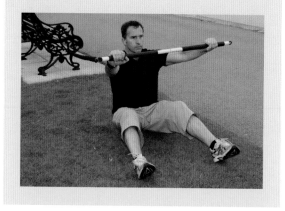

Starting position and action

- Begin standing laterally with your right side closest to the anchor point.
- Hold the lever bar in both hands with your right hand uppermost and the resistance cord at the top of the bar.
- Brace your abdominals and lift the bar to shoulder height as you rotate to your left away from the anchor point, and in a 'chopping wood' action, take the lever bar up and over your head and then slightly down. The movement is not dissimilar to the casting action when fishing.
- Slowly and under control, return the lever bar following the same movement arc back to the start position as you rotate back to your right.
- Repeat the full 'chopping action' with rotations for 15–20 repetitions before changing grip and holding so that your left hand is over your right and you are facing the opposite direction with the anchor point to your left.
- Repeat the chopping action with rotations, yet this time you are rotating to your right as you lift the bar over your shoulders, for 15–20 repetitions.

Starting position and action

- Sit down on the ground holding the lever bar to your chest with the resistance cord to your right and the anchor point behind you.
- With your legs slightly bent, sit upright and engage your abdominals as you press the lever bar away from your chest, keeping your torso relatively still.
- Repeat chest press 15–20 times with the cord to your right before changing the grip position and holding the lever bar with the bungee cord to your left.

Modifications

- Make this exercise much harder by raising one leg throughout to compromise your balance and stability.
- Alternatively, try sitting on a BOSU or stability ball.

Ex 10.71 TRX® Rip™ Trainer rotational sweeps

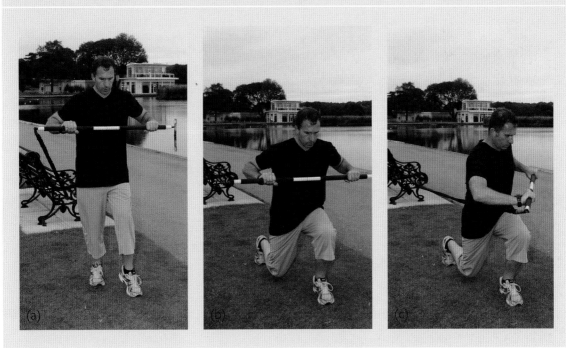

Starting position and action

- Stand facing away from the anchor point, holding on to the lever bar with both hands, with the resistance cord at the end of the bar and to your right side.
- Keeping your abdominals braced, take three quick steps forwards, leading with your left while holding the lever bar, and on the third step, lunge and rotate your torso to your left.
- This sweeping action while holding the lever bar is a complicated movement but similar to taking a run-up and hitting a hockey ball.
- On completion, slowly rotate back and control your movement as you step back to the start.
- Repeat this 'run up and sweep' action 15–20 times before changing the grip so that the resistance cord is to your left.
- Repeat the three step run-up starting with your right leg this time and, holding the lever bar, rotate or 'sweep' to your right side.
- Control the return movement and repeat 15–20 times.

Modifications

- Step/run directly away from the anchor point or at a diagonal or even horizontal to the anchor point for more challenging lateral torque/forces.
- This sweep action can be performed without the run-up, with your feet in a neutral or split stance.

Ex 10.72 TRX® Rip™ Trainer canoe paddles

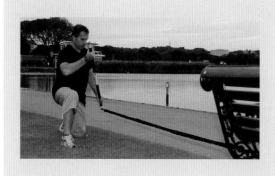

Ex 10.73 TRX® Rip™ Trainer kayak rows

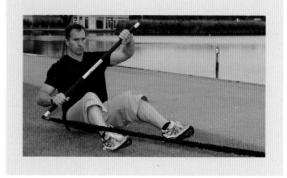

Starting position and action

- Kneel down on your left knee in a half-kneeling position, with your right foot on the ground so as to resemble a canoeing technique with the TRX® Rip™ Trainer secured in front of you.
- Hold the lever bar in both hands with your right hand above your left (when 'paddling' to your left) and keep your abdominals braced.
- The resistance cord should be attached to the bottom of the lever bar.
- Push down with your right hand and pull back with your left in a paddling action, with the lever bar on your left side, and then slowly return back to the start position. Repeat 20–30 times.
- The movement should be controlled yet forceful, with a slower return movement.
- On completion, change your leg and hand position so that you are kneeling on your right knee with your left foot on the ground and have your left hand over your right on the lever bar travelling to your right.
- Repeat paddling action 20–30 times to work the other side, ensuring the resistance cord is at the bottom of the lever.

Starting position and action

- Sit down on the ground holding the lever bar with both hands in front of you at chest height, with the cord to the right end of the bar and the anchor point in front of you.
- Lean back slightly and keep both legs bent.
- Bracing your abdominals, perform a 'figure-8' paddling action so that each end of the lever bar achieves small circles.
- Repeat the 'paddling' action 20–30 times before turning the lever bar around so that the resistance cord is now on your left. Repeat again another 20–30 times.

Modifications

- Place the anchor point behind you to challenge your chest, shoulders and arms. Both positions challenge your core muscles throughout.
- To add difficulty, try raising one leg into the air throughout the paddling actions. Alternatively try sitting on a BOSU with one leg raised.

PUNCH BAG AND POWERBAG DRILLS

When available, punch bags are great in a boot-camp workout as they are heavy, and awkward to carry. Apart from being used as a punch bag and being hit or kicked, they can be lifted, carried, tossed, flipped and thrown in much the same way as Powerbags.

Powerbags are used in training for many sports, with bags varying in weight from 5kg up to 50kg.

Because of their soft but durable nature, and the fact that they are awkward to lift and carry, they are great when used for jumping, throwing and catching drills and any drill that requires you to pick it up and carry it. They are a valuable addition to a personal trainer's 'tool kit' and at costs that don't break the bank, they are certainly an option for the fitness enthusiast.

Ex 10.74 Punch bag straddle squats

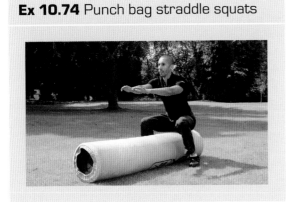

Starting position and action

- Stand upright, straddling a large punch bag, with your knees slightly bent and your abdominals braced.
- Squat down, bending your knees and hips to almost sit on the bag before extending your legs and hips to stand back up, keeping your abdominals braced and spine in neutral.
- Repeat squats on to the punch bag 15–20 times.

Modifications

- Squat and walk so that you squat down to almost touch the bag with your backside, then stand up, take a pace forwards and repeat the squat down as before, repeating along the length of the bag.
- You can squat walk or even squat jump the length of the punch bag. As your buttocks touch the bag, forcefully push off by extending your legs and hips to jump into the air, to land about 0.5m further forwards along the bag.
- Do squat jumps for length of punch bag before turning around and repeating back along the bag. Continue for 20–30 seconds.
- An alternative is to add some upper body force, by squat jumping to one end of the bag, turning around and grabbing the bag with both hands at the end and driving up through your legs, flipping the bag over with your arms, and then running to the start of the bag and straddle jumping along its length.
- At the end, turn around and 'flip' the punch bag before straddle jumping the length of the punch bag again.
- Repeat for 30–60 seconds.
- A further modification is to squat down but to jump and turn 180 degrees, before squatting down and repeating the 180-degree turn back again, repeating 15–20 times.

Ex 10.75 Punch bag shoulder rotations

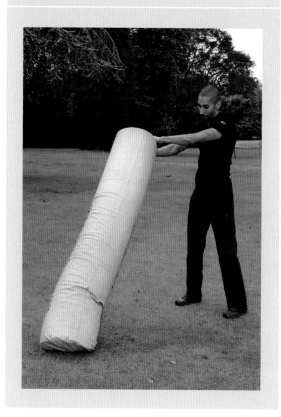

Starting position and action

- This is an excellent core exercise and great for all paddling sports.
- Stand upright, holding the punch bag at one end with both hands, with the base on the ground.
- Keeping your abdominals braced, feet shoulder-width apart and knees bent slightly, hold the end of the punch bag with arms outstretched.
- In this position, with arms slightly bent but tensed, lower the punch bag down to your right side, to almost shoulder height before lifting it back over your head to your left side, again at approximately shoulder height.
- Ensure you are not compromising your body position and that your abdominals are braced throughout.
- The further you lower the punch bag to either side, the greater the resistance and abdominal involvement.
- Repeat 15–30 times before lowering the bag to the floor.

Ex 10.76 Punch bag shoulder carries

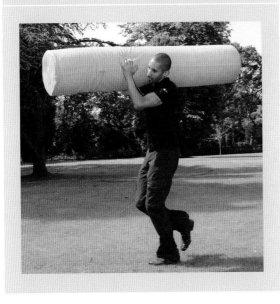

Ex 10.77 Powerbag lift and throws

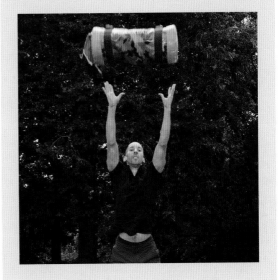

Starting position and action

- Depending upon the size and weight of the punch bag, bend down and place your arms around it, bracing your abdominals fully and using your legs and core strength to lift the punch bag upwards to a vertical position.
- Then squat down to grasp lower down the bag, ready to lift it vertically or tilt it over your shoulder, depending upon size and weight.
- Aim to travel 20–30m holding the punch bag securely.
- Depending upon your fitness level, either walk or run with the punch bag over the distance before placing it down under control.
- This drill can be performed as a relay drill or for individual intervals of 30–60 seconds.

Starting position and action

- Stand with your feet shoulder-width apart and bend your knees to squat down and take hold of the handles of the Powerbag.
- Brace your abdominals as you lift the bag from the floor, extending through your knees and hips powerfully as you pull with your arms to flip the bag over to land on your upper arms.
- From this 'modified hug' position, maintain abdominal tension and partially squat down before extending your legs dynamically as you release the grips, while simultaneously straightening your arms to throw the Powerbag into the air.
- Wherever the bag lands, walk or jog across to it and squat down to hold the handles as before.
- Repeat this dead lift from the floor, flipping the bag on to your upper arms, ready to throw the Powerbag again.
- Repeat 10–15 times.

Ex 10.78 Powerbag reverse tosses

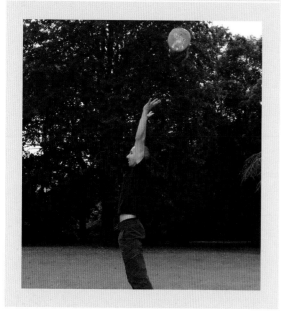

Ex 10.79 Powerbag frontal squats

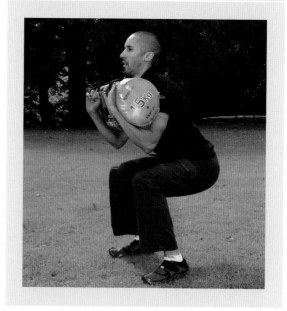

Starting position and action

- With your feet shoulder-width apart, bend your knees and squat down to reach the handles of the Powerbag.
- Take hold of the handles and brace your abdominals as you lift the bag from the floor, extending through your knees and hips powerfully as you pull with your arms to flip the bag over to land on your upper arms.
- Bend your legs, allowing a partial flexion at your hips to lean forward slightly.
- Then push off through your legs, extending your hips and driving your arms upwards to throw the Powerbag into the air over your head to land some distance behind you.
- As the bag lands, turn around and run to it.
- Bend your knees to squat down and take hold of the Powerbag again.
- Repeat the lifts and throws 10–20 times.

Starting position and action

- With your feet shoulder-width apart, bend your knees and squat down to reach the handles of the Powerbag.
- Take hold of the handles and brace your abdominals as you lift the bag from the floor, extending through your knees and hips powerfully as you pull with your arms to flip the bag over to land on your upper arms.
- From this position, keeping your torso upright, squat down, bending your knees to lower until your thighs are almost parallel to the floor.
- Pause briefly at this lowered position, before returning back to a standing position, pushing through your quads and glutes.
- Ensure you do not lean forwards as you squat but keep the body upright, with eyes facing forwards.
- Repeat 15–20 times.

Ex 10.80 Powerbag clean and presses

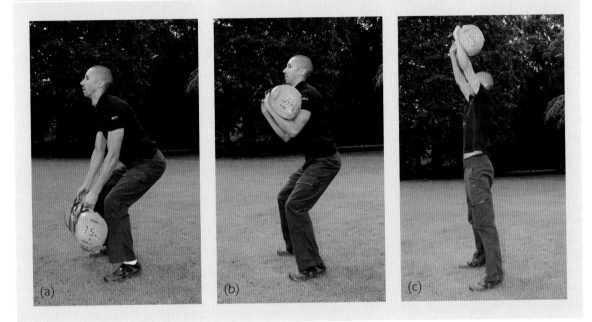

(a)   (b)   (c)

Starting position and action

- Stand behind a Powerbag, with your knees bent and feet shoulder-width apart.
- Squat down by bending your knees and reach forward to grab both handles of the Powerbag.
- Brace your abdominals and, holding the handles of the Powerbag, sit back and lift it with your arms in a clean-and-press action, pulling the bag towards your chest as you drive up with your legs and lift with your arms to flip the bag over to rest on your upper arms.
- From this position, push the Powerbag upwards above your head by extending your arms and, if necessary, assisting the lift with your legs by partially squatting and then driving upwards, extending your legs.
- From the overhead position, lower the Powerbag to your chest to the clean position with your bag resting on your arms, and then lower your arms to drop the bag to the floor.
- Repeat this clean-and-press action 10–15 times.

EXAMPLE BOOTCAMP WORKOUTS

Below are some examples of workout plans that can be used in an outdoor bootcamp, together with several sports-related plans using exercises from this and previous chapters. The sports plans are designed to complement an outdoor workout regime and include specific conditioning exercises and drills that might be of benefit for a sport. These programmes are by no means a sports-specific training plan, merely a guide, identifying muscles and actions used and exercises that might be of benefit.

Table 10.1	Bootcamp workout 1: basic circuit			
Ex no.	**Page**	**Exercise**	**Repetitions**	**Circuit**
Warm-up	14–27	Warm-up variations (see chapter 3)		
10.2	144	Escape drills	30–45 sec	1/16
10.56	189	Suspended atomic push-ups	10–20	2/17
10.57	190	Suspended single-arm power pulls with rotation	10–20	3/18
10.4	145	Piggy-back races	30–45 sec	4/19
10.35	170	ViPR body pushes	5–10	5/20
10.34	170	ViPR body pulls	5–10	6/21
10.8	148	Cone drills	30–45 sec	7/22
10.47	180	Single-arm kettlebell clean and rack	15–20	8/23
10.32	168	ViPR uppercut lunges	15–20	9/24
9.1	115	Step sprints	5–10 sprints	10/25
10.54	187	Kettlebell push-ups with row	15–25	11/26
10.51	184	Kettlebell Turkish get-ups	5–10	12/27
10.19	157	Tyre pulling	5–10 sprints	13/28
10.77	205	Powerbag lift and throws	10–15	14/29
10.69	200	TRX® Rip™ Trainer axe chops	15–25	15 /30
	237–40	Cool-down and stretch		

Table 10.2	Bootcamp workout 2: interval circuit and giant-set circuit			
Ex No.	**Page**	**Exercise**	**Option 1 interval circuit**	**Option 2 giant-set circuit**
Warm-up	14–27	Warm-up variations (see chapter 3)		
10.9	148	Shuttle runs	A1/A16	A1/A6/A11
10.44	178	Kettlebell swings	A2/A17	A2/A7/A12
10.52	185	Kettlebell halos	A3/A18	A3/A8/A13
10.21	159	Hitting tyre with sledgehammer	A4/A19	A4/A9/A14
10.16	154	Farmer's walk with spare tyres	A5/A20	A5/A10/A15
10.33	169	ViPR uppercuts to block	A6/A21	B1/B7
10.19	157	Tyre pulling	A7/A22	B2/B8
10.79	206	Powerbag frontal squats	A8/A23	B3/B9
10.60 10.61	193	Suspended T/Y deltoid raises	A/A24	B4/B10
10.18	156	Tyre flipping	A10/A25	B5/B11
10.70	200	TRX® Rip™ Trainer seated chest presses	A11/A26	B6/B12
10.71	201	TRX® Rip™ Trainer rotational sweeps	A12/A27	C1/C5/C9
10.30	166	ViPR lateral flip drills	A13/A28	C2/ C6/C10
10.58	191	Suspended total body burpees	A14/A29	C3/C7/C11
10.31	167	ViPR integrated clean and press with lunge	A15/A30	C4/ C8/C12
	237–40	Cool-down and stretch		

Table 10.3		Bootcamp workout 3: Alternative circuit and giant-set circuit		
Ex no.	**Page**	**Exercise**	**Option 1 circuit**	**Option 2 giant-set circuit**
Warm-up	14–27	Warm-up variations (*see* chapter 3)		
10.23	160	BOSU walk-downs	A1/A16	A1/A6/A11
10.41	175	ViPR ice skater	A2/A17	A2/A7/A12
10.67	198	TRX® Rip™ Trainer squats to asymmetric press	A3/A18	A3/A8/A13
10.65	196	TRX® Rip™ Trainer squats to high row	A4/A19	A4/A9/A14
10.38	172	ViPR 'thread the needle'	A5/A20	A5/A10/A15
10.56	189	Suspended atomic push-ups	A6/A21	B1/B7
10.78	206	Powerbag reverse tosses	A7/A22	B2/B8
10.62	194	Suspended dynamic lunges	A8/A23	B3/B9
10.80	207	Powerbag clean and presses	A9/A24	B4/B10
10.57	190	Suspended single-arm power pulls with rotation	A10/A25	B5/B11
10.76	205	Punch bag shoulder carries	A11/A26	B6/B12
10.21	159	Hitting tyre with sledgehammer	A12/A27	C1/C5/C9
10.20	158	Tyre lift/pull-downs	A13/A28	C2/C6/C10
10.18	156	Tyre flipping	A14/A29	C3/C7/C11
10.16	154	Farmer's walk with spare tyres	A15/A30	C4/C8/C12
	237–40	Cool-down and stretch		

Table 10.4	Sports drills workout (various sports)			
Ex no.	**Page**	**Exercise**	**Option 1 circuit**	**Option 2 circuit**
Warm-up	14–27	Warm-up variations (see chapter 3)		
10.8	148	Cone drills	A1/A16	A1/A6/A11
10.13	152	Cone co-ordination srills	A2/A17	A2/A7/A12
10.12	151	Bungee-cord-resisted sprints	A3/A18	A3/A8/A13
10.22	159	Sled pushing	A4/A19	A4/A9/A14
10.11	150	Bungee-cord-assisted sprints	A5/A20	A5/A10/A15
10.53	186	Kettlebell clean and rack on BOSU	A6/A21	B1/B7
9.6	119	Medicine ball power throws to floor	A7/A22	B2/B8
10.49	182	Single-arm snatch and squats	A8/A23	B3/B9
10.52	185	Kettlebell halos (on BOSU)	A9/A24	B4/B10
10.77	205	Powerbag lift and throws	A10/A25	B5/B11
9.7	120	Kneeling oblique throws	A11A26	B6/B12
10.65	196	TRX® Rip™ Trainer squats to high row	A12/A27	C1/C5/C9
10.66	197	TRX® Rip™ Trainer squats to low row	A13/A28	C2/C6/C10
10.69	200	TRX® Rip™ Trainer axe chops	A14/A29	C3/C7/C11
10.71	201	TRX® Rip™ Trainer rotational sweeps	A15/A30	C4/C8/C12
	237–40	Cool-down and stretch		

Table 10.5		Hiking/running workout		
Ex no.	Page	Exercise	Option 1 circuit	Option 2 giant-set circuit
Warm-up	14–27	Warm-up variations (see chapter 3)		
10.54	187	Kettlebell push-ups with row	A1/A16	A1/A6/A11
10.23	160	BOSU walk-downs	A2/A17	A2/A7/A12
7.23	72	Single-arm rows	A3/A18	A3/A8/A13
7.32	80	Step-ups to balance with overhead press	A4/A19	A4/A9/A14
9.12	123	Suspended chest presses	A5/A20	A5/A10/A15
10.22	159	Sled pushing	A6/A21	B1/B7
7.31	79	Lunge and pulls	A7/A22	B2/B8
10.80	207	Powerbag clean and presses	A8/A23	B3/B9
8.32	109	Bounding	A9/A24	B4/B10
8.20	100	Gecko crawl with push-ups	A10/A25	B5/B11
10.41	175	ViPR ice skater	A11/A26	B6/B12
10.77	205	Powerbag lift and throws	A12/A27	C1/C5/C9
8.30	108	Single leg high step-ups	A13/A28	C2/C6/C10
9.10	121	Single-leg balances with lateral flexion	A14/A29	C3/C7/C11
10.16	154	Farmer's walk with spare tyres	A15/A30	C4/C8/C12
	237–40	Cool-down and stretch		

Ex no.	Page	Exercise	Option 1 circuit	Option 2 giant-set circuit
		Table 10.6 Windsurfing/surfing workout		
Warm-up	14–27	Warm-up variations (see chapter 3)		
7.11	64	Stability ball roll-outs	A1/A16	A1/A6/A11
9.25	132	Suspension Training® dynamic lateral squat jumps	A2/A17	A2/A7/A12
10.56	189	Suspended atomic push-ups	A3/A18	A3/A8/A13
8.22	102	Railing pull-ups (feet on a stability ball)	A4/A19	A4/A9/A14
10.37	171	ViPR horizontal drags	A5/A20	A5/A10/A15
10.47	186	Single-arm kettlebell clean and racks (on BOSU)	A6/A21	B1/B7
10.57	190	Suspended single arm power pulls with rotation	A7/A22	B2/B8
10.24	161	BOSU split squats	A8/A23	B3/B9
10.61	193	Suspended Y-deltoid raisees	A9/A24	B4/B10
7.18	69	Single-arm stability ball chest presses	A10/A25	B5/B11
10.69	200	TRX® Rip™ Trainer axe chops	A11/A26	B6/B12
10.62	194	Suspended balanced lunges	A12/A27	C1/C5/C9
10.65	196	TRX® Rip™ Trainer squats to high row	A13/A28	C2/C6/C10
10.25	162	BOSU squat thrusts to balance	A14/A29	C3/C7/C11
8.14	96	Impossible bridges	A15/A30	C4/C8/C12
	237–40	Cool-down and stretch		

Table 10.7	Skiing/snowboarding workout			
Ex no.	Page	Exercise	Option 1 circuit	Option 2 giant-set circuit
Warm-up	14–27	Warm-up variations (see chapter 3)		
10.41	175	ViPR ice skater	A1/A16	A1/A6/A11
7.17	68	Push-ups with rotation	A2/A17	A2/A7/A12
8.33	110	Split lunge jumps	A3/A18	A3/A8/A13
10.57	190	Suspended single-arm power pulls with rotation	A4/A19	A4/A9/A14
8.32	109	Bounding	A5/A20	A5/A10/A15
7.19	70	Stability ball push-ups	A6/A21	B1/B7
10.52	185	Kettlebell halos	A7/A22	B2/B8
9.29	134	Squat jumps with floor touch and rotation	A8/A23	B3 /B9
9.6	119	Medicine ball power throws to floor	A9/ A24	B4 /B10
10.67	198	TRX® Rip™ Trainer squats and asymmetric press	A10/A25	B5/B11
10.14	152	Plyometric cone jumps	A11/A26	B6/B12
10.63	195	Suspended dips	A12/A27	C1/C5/C9
10.15	153	Lateral cone jumps with rotation	A13/A28	C2/C6/C10
10.47	186	Single-arm kettlebell clean and rack (on BOSU)	A14/A29	C3/C7/C11
7.30	78	Side lunges with dumbbell pick-ups	A15/A30	C4/C8/C12
	237–40	Cool-down and stretch		

Table 10.8		Canoeing/kayaking/stand-up paddleboarding workout		
Ex no.	Page	Exercise	Option 1 circuit	Option 2 giant-set circuit
Warm-up	14–27	Warm-up variations (see chapter 3)		
9.6	119	Medicine ball power throws to floor (on BOSU)	A1/A16	A1/A6/A11
10.32	168	ViPR uppercut lunges	A2/A17	A2/A7/A12
9.12	123	Suspended chest presses	A3/A18	A3/A8/A13
10.73	202	TRX® Rip™ Trainer kayak rows	A4/A19	A4/A9/A14
10.24	161	BOSU split squats	A5/A20	A5/A10/A15
10.52	185	Kettlebell halos (on BOSU)	A6/A21	B1/B7
10.72	202	TRX® Rip™ Trainer canoe paddles	A7/A22	B2/B8
10.26	163	BOSU dynamic lateral push-ups	A8/A23	B3/B9
8.22	102	Railing pull-ups (feet on BOSU)	A9/A24	B4/B10
8.7	92	Resistance tube woodchop (on BOSU)	A10/A25	B5/B11
10.40	174	ViPR squat and sweeps	A11/A26	B6/B12
10.67	198	TRX® Rip™ Trainer squats to assymetric press	A12/A27	C1/C5/C9
10.28	164	BOSU Russian twists	A13/A28	C2/C6/C10
10.54	187	Kettlebell push-ups with row	A14/A29	C3/C7/C11
10.64	195	Suspended supine hip presses	A15/A30	C4/C8/C12
	237–40	Cool-down and stretch		

Kayaking: Perform exercises in seated position on a BOSU where appropriate

Canoeing: Perform exercises in kneeling position on a BOSU where appropriate

Paddleboarding: Perform exercise standing up on a BOSU where appropriate

// TRIM TRAILS

11

When working as a freelance personal trainer in south-west London in the early 1990s, I remember seeing an early trim trail in Battersea Park, and although it was only a few logs, beams and climbing bars laid out in a specific order over a relatively small area, it was a feature within the park. I remember taking clients there and on numerous occasions using the trail as an opportunist exercise feature. While I am not suggesting that this was the first trim trail, it was the first I had seen that was effective.

Trim trails and commercial play zones have popped up in numerous parks and public spaces in recent years and I think it is great that there is an attempt by councils and local government to address fitness issues and the health of the nation by creating opportunities for exercise in the open. However, I am often surprised by the questionable exercise equipment choices that I have found in some parks. I have my own opinions on what is effective, yet I am sure that providing the opportunity for unsupervised exercise brings with it some problems and potential risks. Unfortunately, while in many parks there could have been a fantastic investment in inexpensive trim trail fitness apparatus, all too often the 'safety police' have taken control and consequently the equipment is generally ineffective for the majority of fitness levels, more a token gesture rather than a real opportunity for sustained activity and exercise. Trim trails need to represent the needs of the community as a whole, providing a suitable challenge for all fitness levels. While a few companies on the market have got the right idea, from what I have seen in my travels, not every council grasps the concept of effective overload for achieving a fitness gain.

Exercise, and any activity that requires you to balance, jump, leap or climb, involves risk, yet, within reason, that is how the body develops – by utilising environments that are physically challenging, dealing with these challenges and overcoming them in a learned fashion. The best trim trails should combine the fascination of imaginative play from our childhood together with the specific physical challenges of working different muscles. The design should embrace the environment, rather than stick out like a purple plastic sore thumb.

My personal favourite trim-trail equipment is largely wood-based but includes ropes, foot bridges, beams and climbing nets and ladders. Such equipment can:

- challenge your balance (rope bridge/Burma bridge, wobble boards, stepping stones, balance beams);
- increase your heart rate and agility through jumping, leaping, climbing or stepping on to or over the equipment (log vaults, hurdles, scramble/commando nets);

- provide a basis for bodyweight exercises to increase strength and co-ordination (monkey bars/pull-up bars, beams, parallel dip bars).

Below are some examples of effective trim-trail exercises to train your cardiovascular fitness, balance, co-ordination, strength, power and agility.

Ex 11.1 Balance beams

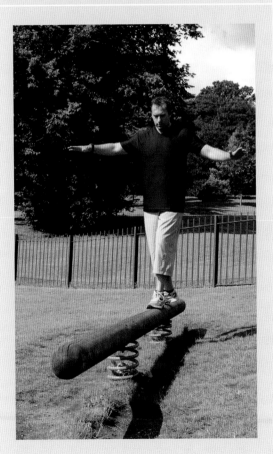

Starting position and action

- Step up on to the low-level balance beam, one foot at a time, using your arms to assist your balance.
- Then slowly walk along the balance beam, maintaining your balance throughout.
- As you progress, increase your speed.

Modifications

- To challenge your balance further, try walking forwards and then backwards along the balance beam.
- Alternatively, try turning around 180 degrees and walking back along the beam.
- You could add jumps or even jump-turns, but this requires excellent balance and co-ordination. Only try this when you are proficient with regular walking and turning actions.

Ex 11.2 Log hurdles

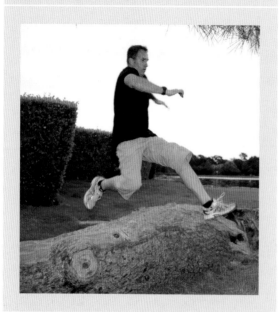

Ex 11.3 Burma/rope bridges

(a)

(b)

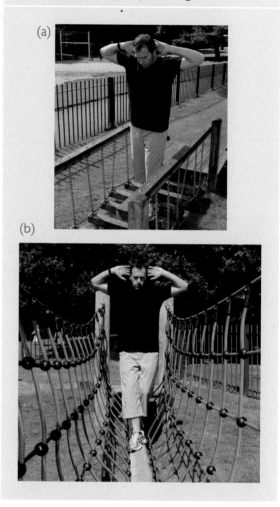

Starting position and action

- If you find a fallen tree, large branch, park bench, bush or anything that you feel confident that you can jump over, give yourself plenty of run-up space and try to hurdle over it.
- Before trying to run and jump over the obstacle, always make sure you can clearly see the landing area and check that it is safe to jump over.
- Also, when jumping over large obstacles, such as bushes or fallen trees, always be aware of loose branches or twigs that could hinder your jump.
- This dynamic exercise creates an energetic interval that challenges your co-ordination, power and fitness level, especially if you try and repeat the jumps 5–10 times.

Starting position and action

- Hold on to the guide ropes and step on to the rope bridge one foot at a time.
- Use the guide ropes for balance but try not to hang on too tight.
- Aim to cross the bridge under control yet with confidence in your stepping action.
- When confident, try and maintain your balance walking without holding the guide ropes at all.

Ex 11.4 Stepping stones

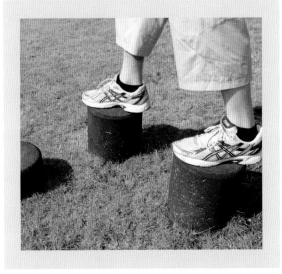

Starting position and action

- Stand behind the row of steps or mini tree stumps and then step up on to the first one, maintaining your balance.
- Depending upon the gap between the stepping stones, step or leap from one to the next, cushioning your landing through your knees.
- When you are balanced, continue to the end, then turn around and repeat again.

Ex 11.5 Sprung wobble boards

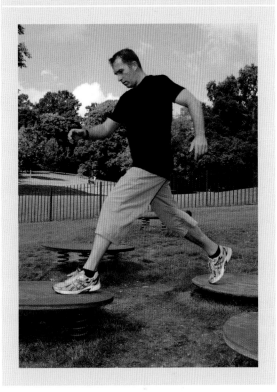

Starting position and action

- Wobble boards are a relatively safe way of challenging your balance as they are sprung and so are naturally self-righting, yet as you move across them they tilt according to your bodyweight and foot placement.
- Try challenging your balance by stepping or jumping on to these boards, controlling your body movement and alignment as you land.
- You could perform various squat jumps and jump-turns or use a resistance tube and perform specific conditioning exercises, such as lateral raises, single-arm curls and presses, etc.

Ex 11.6 Decline bench reverse curls

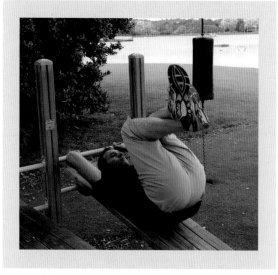

Ex 11.7 Incline bench abdominal curls

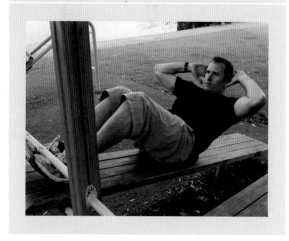

If you see an incline or decline bench, a number of exercises can be performed on the same bench, depending upon your fitness level.

Starting position and action

- Lie face up with your head to the top of the bench, holding on to the top of the bench or support bar with both hands.
- Flex your hips and knees and hold your legs up, maintaining tension through your abdominals.
- In this position, contract your abdominals and curl your thighs towards your chest in a slow movement, lifting your buttocks and lower back off the floor.
- Hold this contracted position with your thighs drawn into your chest and then lower your legs back to the start position.
- Repeat these reverse abdominal curls 12–20 times.

Starting position and action

- Lie face up on the incline bench with your feet hooked underneath the support bar.
- With hands forwards, across your chest or behind your head, brace your abdominals and slowly curl upwards.
- Lift your upper and mid-back off the bench as you curl your chest towards your hips, lifting about 25–30cm with your knees bent.
- Pause briefly in the curled position and then lower back to the bench.
- Repeat incline curls 12–20 times.

Ex 11.8 Railing vaults

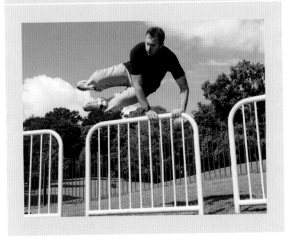

Ex 11.9 Monkey bars

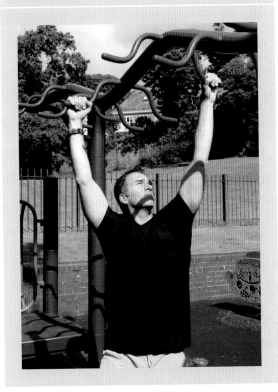

Starting position and action

- Grip a railing with both hands and with your feet on one side.
- Push off your legs and stabilise your body with your arms as you brace your abdominals and jump over the railing to land with both feet together on the other side.
- Cushion your landing by bending your knees and then rapidly extend your legs to jump back over the railing to land where you started.
- Repeat jumps, keeping your abdominals braced for 30–50 seconds.

Modifications

- Depending upon the design of the railings, the number and relative heights you can perform over and under techniques whereby you can hurdle or jump over the bars and then crawl or clamber underneath for increased fitness and agility training.
- Aim to jump over one hurdle and under the next repeating for 30–50 seconds, before resting.

Starting position and action

- Jump up to grab hold of the monkey bars with both hands.
- Keep your knees slightly bent and hips partially flexed to help assist your 'grappling' movement.
- Keeping your abdominals braced and arms slightly bent, partially pull yourself up so as to be able to reach the next monkey bar.
- As carefully as you can, swing and reach to the next bar alternating hands as you traverse the bars.

Ex 11.10 Chin-ups

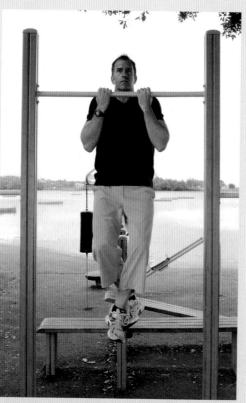

Modification

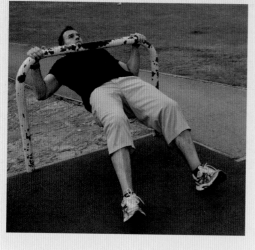

Starting position and action

- Hang from a chin-up bar at arms' length with your palms facing you.
- Contract your biceps to try and lift your body upwards so that your chin is over the bar.
- From this top position, drop down slowly by eccentrically contracting your biceps muscles.
- The full chin-up is a very advanced exercise and so do as many repetitions as you can comfortably manage.

Modifications

- For those of you who are strong enough to perform full chin-ups, try varying your hand position so that your palms are facing away from you. With your palms facing away from you, you could also try a wide-grip position.
- If you cannot perform the full chin-up, try using a step to help you push off.
- In this position try and lower yourself as slowly as you can, working the biceps muscles eccentrically until your arms are fully extended and you are in the full hanging position.
- Repeat these 'negative' chin-ups 5–15 times as a training aid for strengthening the relative muscles so as to perform full chin-ups when you have developed greater strength.
- If no high bar is available or if negative pull-ups are too challenging, why not try the assisted pull up from a railing.

Ex 11.11 Parallel bars dips

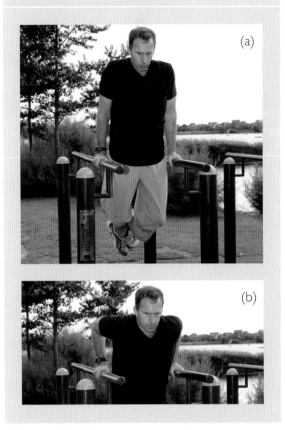

(a)

(b)

Ex 11.12 Commando net climbs

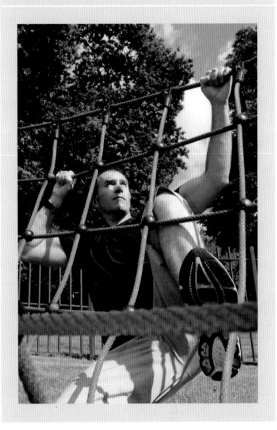

Starting position and action

- Lift yourself up on to the parallel bars by jumping up and supporting your bodyweight through your arms and shoulders.
- In this supported position, keeping your abdominals braced, lower down by bending your arms and flexing your elbows to almost 90 degrees.
- Push back up to the extended arm start position, contracting your triceps.
- As you bend your arms, lean forwards to keep your forearms vertical before pushing back to an upright position.
- Repeat 10–20 times.

Starting position and action

- If you are lucky enough to have a commando net on your trim trail, this is a fantastic piece of equipment to simply climb up by any means possible.
- Take a run and jump on to the net and then clamber up it, arm by arm until you reach the top of the frame.
- Climb up at a speed that you can maintain until you have reached the top and then swing your legs over to the other side and carefully climb back down.

BUGGY WORKOUTS

12

Buggy workouts, i.e. exercising with your child in their pushchair, have seen a huge rise in interest in recent years, partly due to the development of improved pushchairs and the realisation, largely from personal trainers, that there is a target market out there of mums whose time constraints and childcare concerns can be overcome through park or beach workouts with your child either on a one-to-one basis or in a group environment.

Many of these 'buggy' franchises have been developed by self-styled fitness enthusiasts who have had positive results following the birth of their baby and wanted to share this enthusiasm with other mothers. These programmes are not only a great opportunity for socialising with others mums and interacting with your baby, but you are getting a workout as well. In some cases this franchise concept has gone national, with many personal trainers and/or young mums buying into a brand to deliver interactive workouts in parks, commons and open spaces.

Whether you are signed up to a franchise or, as a personal trainer, you want to set up your own buggy workout, the bottom line is that the workout should follow a safe and structured progressive programme of interactive exercises that involves mother and child, whether visually or by verbal or physical interaction. The majority of buggy workout programmes I have observed and researched are fundamentally safe and effective, and do provide opportunities for progression.

The exercises used are by no means fixed – it really is down to your own imagination (within reason) or that of the trainer running the session. Because you are working with minimal equipment, it can be stored or carried in your buggy. There are many bodyweight exercises in this book so you could apply a selection from the beach, garden or park workout

If you are considering your own buggy workout – whether on your own, with a friend in a park environment or on a personal trainer-led programme – there are a few important aspects to consider. Firstly, it is not wise to start working out until you have had your six-week postnatal check and your doctor is happy for you to exercise. It is fine in the build-up to the six-week check for you to begin walking with your child, but take things gently at first. If you have had a Caesarean then the guideline is 10–12 weeks before moderately intense exercise but again, always check with your doctor.

As with any exercise programme, ensure you perform a graduated warm-up and mobilise and dynamically stretch the muscles and joints (*see* chapter 3). If you are new to exercise or unsure of what to do, you might find that joining a class is the better option initially. This way, the qualified instructor will take you safely through the warm-up process and guide you through the exercise selection without you having to think of suitable exercises.

If you were a relatively accomplished exerciser prior to the birth of your baby, the rule of thumb when starting back is to follow a warm-up that gradually raises your heart rate followed by mobility exercises and some dynamic stretches, remembering that any exercise you choose should be at a lower level than you were once able to perform. After all, it might have been almost a year since you stopped exercising and you should take things easy to begin with.

Within this chapter, I have identified exercises that might be suitable for a mother of low to moderate fitness who is easing herself back into

shape following the birth of her baby, whether this be soon after her six-week check-up or is she hasn't shifted the weight and her little one has just seen their first birthday.

Below are some exercises used in a buggy workout that train the major muscle groups. If performed regularly, they will help you to achieve fat loss, improved fitness and better tone, all relative to your dietary intake. You won't need a special buggy for these workouts – as long as your child is comfortable and happy and the handles are at the right height, you are fine to use your regular pushchair.

Above all, as long as you enjoy the session, your child appears happy you get moderately hot and sweaty, burn a few calories and do a few conditioning exercises, the workout will be of benefit. As with all activity, circumstance, environment, ability and enjoyment level all need to balance out to achieve a positive result.

Ex 12.1 Speed walk intervals

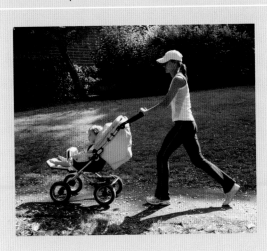

Starting position and action

- Hold the buggy handle with a firm grip and begin walking at a reasonable pace.
- Maintaining an upright posture and without locking your arms, increase your walking speed to a power walk so that you are pushing off your toes with each step.
- Continue this fast-paced walk for 30–50m before slowing down slightly to a more comfortable speed for 20–50m.
- Repeat this fast walk/comfortable walk interval over a distance of 500m to 1km.

Ex 12.2 Forward lunges to buggy press

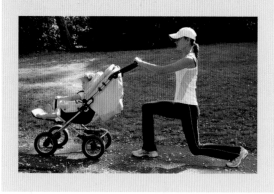

Starting position and action

- Stand behind the buggy, holding it by the handle with your feet hip-distance apart, and in an upright posture, with your spine in neutral alignment.
- Step forwards into a lunge with your right foot while simultaneously pushing your buggy forward a stride length.
- As your front thigh lowers to almost parallel with the floor, with your knee bent to 90 degrees, push back off your right leg, contracting your thigh and buttock muscles to push yourself back to a standing position.
- Ensure you use sufficient force during this push as you will have both your bodyweight and the weight of the buggy to deal with.
- From the standing position, decelerate the buggy with your arms, keeping your abdominals braced, and then step forwards, this time with your left leg as you push the buggy away a stride length, as before.
- Lower down until your left thigh draws parallel to the floor before pushing back to a standing position, pulling the buggy with you.

Ex 12.3 Single-arm chest presses

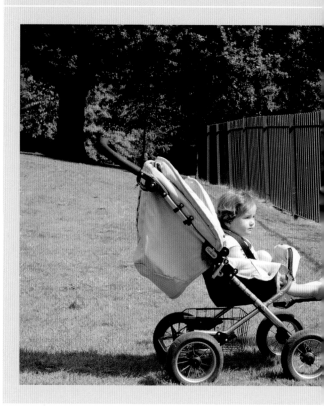

Starting position and action

- Secure a resistance tube around a post or bench and hold both handles in your right hand.
- Stand facing away from the anchor point in a staggered stance with your left leg forwards and both knees slightly bent, holding the handles near your right shoulder, elbow behind you and your palm facing down.
- The resistance tube should be under partial tension.
- Bracing your abdominals, slowly press the resistance tube forwards in front of your chest, ensuring you are not leaning or using your bodyweight to assist the movement.

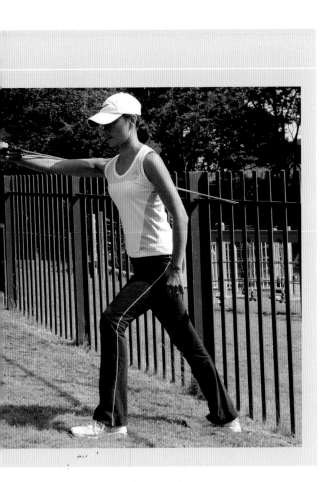

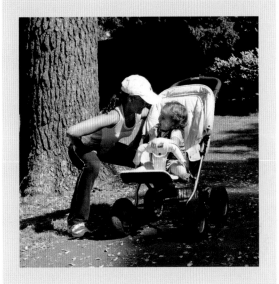

Ex 12.4 Peak-a-boo squats

- Pause briefly in the extended position, ensuring your back remains stabilised, then slowly return to the start position.
- It is important not to lean back during this exercise as this reduces the stabilisation effect – always use the correct resistance, even reducing the resistance but adding repetitions to ensure quality of movement and stabilisation.
- Repeat 12–15 times.

Modification

- To increase the stabilisation required, this exercise can be performed in a kneeling position.

Starting position and action

- Stand to the side of the buggy, just out of sight of your child, with your feet shoulder-width apart, facing the buggy.
- Dynamically step out to your side, dropping into a lateral squat to the front of the buggy so that you can see your child and they can see you.
- As you squat down, keep your torso upright and bend through your knees and hips to sit into a lateral squat so that you can play 'peek-a-boo' with your child.
- After completing any interaction while in the squat position, push off your leg to return back to a standing position.
- Repeat for 10–15 lateral squats leading with one side before moving to the other side of the buggy and repeating, stepping out with your other leg.

Ex 12.5 Leg abductions holding buggy

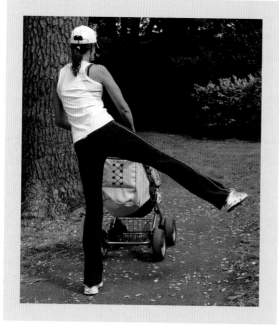

Ex 12.6 Mulberry bush lateral squats

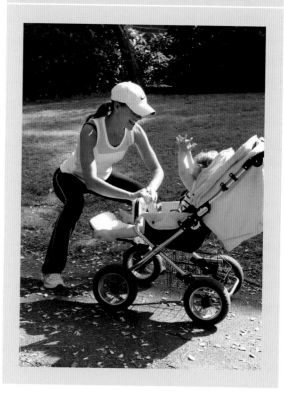

Starting position and action

- Stand behind your buggy, with your palms resting lightly on the handles for balance.
- Stand with your feet hip-distance apart, with a neutral spine and upright posture.
- Move your weight over to your left leg and with the knee slightly bent, lift your right leg out to the side.
- Aim to laterally abduct your right leg, lifting it about 1m from the start position and about 0.5m from the floor, with your toes pointing forwards throughout.
- Keep your abdominals braced and maintain an upright posture without leaning either forwards or to the side. Repeat lifting and lowering your right leg for 20–30 repetitions, before lowering your leg and repeating on the other side.

Starting position and action

- This is a child-interaction drill and is just as much about engaging with your toddler as it is about your own exercise.
- Face your child at the front of the buggy then step into a lateral squat by stepping out to your right and squatting down.
- Continue this lateral squatting action, stepping out with your right leg and then bringing your left leg in to return to a standing position until you have completely circled the buggy.
- Repeat squatting, this time in the other direction, leading with your left leg, still facing the buggy and laterally squatting around the buggy to your left.

- Repeat three full circles in each direction.

Modifications

- Instead of laterally squatting around the buggy you could always perform a lateral side-step or shuffling action, facing the buggy all the time.
- On completing a full circle either change direction or continue for two or three circles before changing direction.
- Repeat for a total of 15–20 full 'buggy circles'.

Ex 12.7 Park bench push-ups

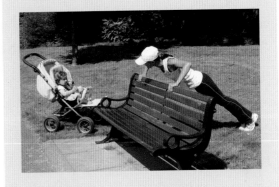

Starting position and action

- Stand behind a park bench and place your hands on the upright back rest of the bench about one and a half times' shoulder-width apart so that your arms are perpendicular to your torso and your legs are extended behind you.
- With your weight going through your arms and shoulders, brace your abdominals and bend your arms to lower your chest to the bench before extending your arms and pushing through your shoulders and chest to return to the extended arm position.
- Repeat 12–20 times.

Modifications

- To increase the intensity, perform the push-up with your hands on the seat of the bench as this will put more of your weight through your arms and chest.
- To intensify this drill further you could try an advanced incline push-up with your feet on the bench and your hands on the ground. This is an intense exercise, so ensure your abdominals are fully braced and do not let your back sag at any stage.

Ex 12.8 Kneeling shoulder presses

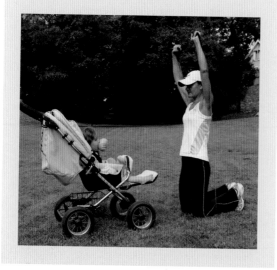

Ex 12.9 Interval buggy sprints

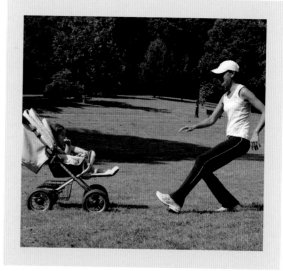

Starting position and action

- Kneel on a resistance tube, in an upright position with your hips in neutral and your feet together behind you.
- Hold the resistance tube by its handles at your shoulders with your palms facing away from you.
- Keeping your abdominals braced, push the handles upwards over your head so that your hands almost touch, with your arms extended.
- Pause briefly in this top position and then lower your hands slowly back to the start position by your shoulders.
- Repeat 12–20 times, making sure you maintain correct alignment through your torso.

Modification

- To intensify this exercise, you can hold both handles in one hand and perform a single-arm shoulder press, making sure you do not lean over to one side to assist the movement.

Starting position and action

- Stand 20–30m in front of your buggy, facing your child so that they can see you.
- With your feet hip-distance apart in a staggered stance with knees slightly bent, accelerate in a sprinting action towards your buggy for 10–15m, yet decelerate over the last 5m to end proximal to your buggy and child.
- Any vocal interaction while running to capture your child's interest is purely optional – but any kind of 'Wheeeeeeee!' or 'Where's Mummy? Here I am!' wouldn't go amiss!
- Upon reaching the buggy, accelerate backwards to the start point, while still engaging with your child.
- Repeat these forward and backward sprints for 6–10 complete repetitions, before resting.

Ex 12.10 Triceps kickbacks

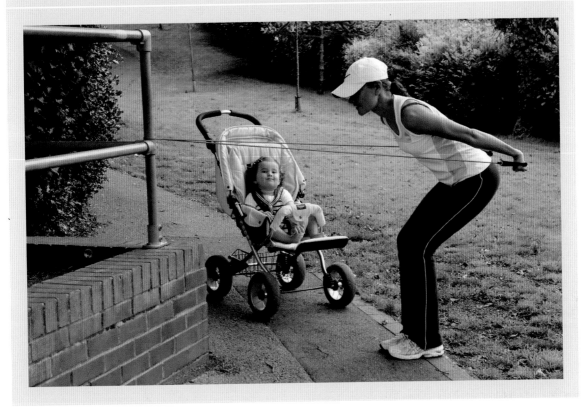

Starting position and action

- Wrap a resistance tube around a railing or post and stand back to create tension on the resistance tube, while facing the post.
- Keeping your abdominals braced with feet either hip-distance apart or in a partial split-stance, lean forwards from your waist, keeping your elbows close to your ribs, with hands forwards, holding the grips in a fully flexed arm position.
- From this leaning forwards position while maintaining abdominal tension and bent legs, pull the handles back, keeping your upper arms still by contracting your triceps fully to bring your arms to a near locked position, with hands behind your elbows.
- Pause briefly when your triceps are fully contracted and then slowly return your hands to the starting flexed arm position, keeping your upper arms parallel to the floor and elbows fixed.
- Repeat 15–30 times.

Modifications

- This exercise can be completed starting with palms facing down (pronated grip) or facing up (supinated).

EXAMPLE BUGGY WORKOUT

The buggy workout can incorporate numerous options from the garden, beach, park and boot-camp chapters according to fitness level, number of participants and equipment used. Below is an example using minimal equipment (only body-weight and a resistance tube).

Ex no.	Page	Exercise	Buggy workout interval circuit
Warm-up	14–27	Warm-up variations (see chapter 3)	
12.1	225	Speed walk intervals	A1/A16
12.2	226	Forward lunges to buggy press	A2/A17
12.7	229	Park bench push-ups	A3/A18
8.22	102	Railing pull-ups	A4/A19
12.4	227	Peek-a-boo squats	A5/A20
12.8	230	Kneeling shoulder presses	A6/A21
12.5	228	Leg abductions holding buggy	A7/A22
12.9	230	Interval buggy sprints	A8/A23
7.5	60	Abdominal bridges	A9/A24
12.10	231	Triceps kickbacks	A10/A25
7.34	82	Hip thrusts	A11/A26
7.36	83	Biceps curls	A12/A27
12.3	226	Single-arm chest presses	A13/A28
12.6	228	Mulberry bush lateral squats	A14/A29
7.7	61	Supermans	A15/A30
	237–40	Cool-down and stretch	

Table 12.1 Buggy workout

APPENDIX 1:
SELF-MYOFASCIAL RELEASE

If a muscle is tight or weak it can have an impact on your overall training, since if it is not rectified through stretching or specific strengthening exercises, it can create a muscular imbalance that can ultimately affect your performance, posture and natural movement. Tight muscles need to return to their normal length for optimum performance and often this can be a gradual approach

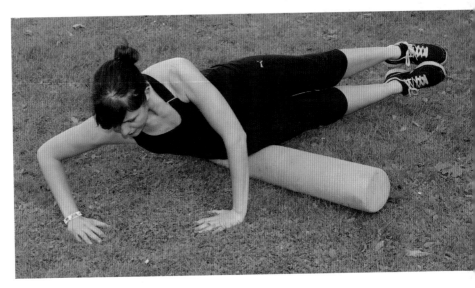

of stretching techniques, re-alignment and re-educating the muscle of its correct purpose.[24] While static and dynamic stretches can assist the flexibility of a joint by helping to stretch a muscle, *self-myofascial release (SMR)* is considered to be one of the most effective ways to assist flexibility.

SMR requires a pressure to follow the line of the muscle and can be used to assist releasing a particularly tight muscle prior to activity, in addition to

other dynamic stretches.[25] SMR techniques can help to 'iron out' a tight muscle and can help to restore normal muscle length. Usually you will use a *foam roller*. Place this under the relevant muscle. Slowly and gently roll over the foam roller, pausing for 20–30 seconds where you might encounter any tight spots, applying pressure as you roll. As well as stretching out the muscle, this stimulates the *Golgi tendon organ*, which assists in allowing the muscle tightness to be reduced.

If you are aware of tight muscles or stiff, inflexible joints, before embarking on a training programme it is worth seeking out a reputable trainer who can offer advice on any muscle imbalance you might have and structure a workout around your specific needs and requirements.

Self-myofascial release benefits
- Neuromuscular efficiency
- Can improve flexibility about a specific joint
- Reduces muscle soreness
- Corrects muscle imbalances

SMR STRETCHES

Gastrocnemius

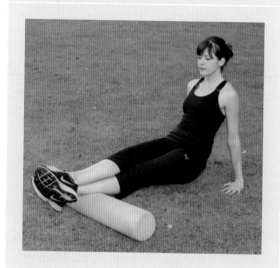

Hamstrings

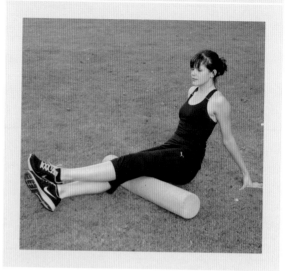

Starting position and action

- Sit on the floor with your left ankle resting on the foam roller and cross your right leg on to your left ankle to increase the pressure.
- Lift your hips up by supporting your bodyweight on your arms and gently 'walk' yourself down towards the foam roller so that it rolls slowly towards your knee.

Starting position and action

- Sit on the floor with the foam roller under your right knee and cross your left leg over your right to intensify the stretch to your right leg.
- Support your bodyweight with your arms and gently move yourself forwards so that the foam roller travels up towards your hip.

Quads

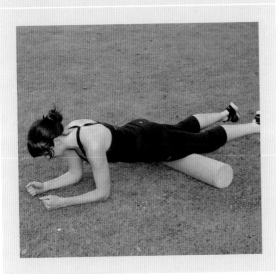

Piriformis

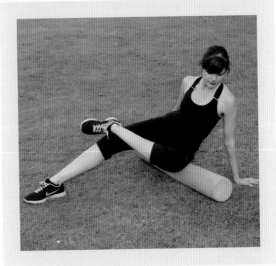

Starting position and action

- Lie face down with your thigh over the foam roller, with your arms supporting your body-weight.
- Gently roll across the foam roller so that it travels from your pelvic bone down to your knee, remembering to keep the roller towards the outside of your thigh.

Starting position and action

- Begin in a seated position on the foam roller with your left leg crossed over your right knee and your bodyweight supported through your arms.
- Roll the foam roller across the outside of the hip area, just above the gluteal area.

Iliotibial (IT) band

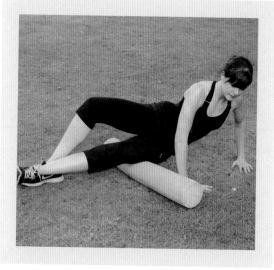

Tensor fascia latae

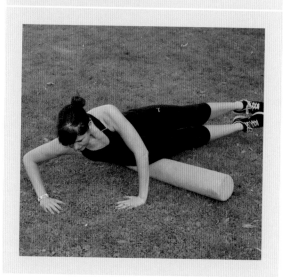

Starting position and action

- Position yourself on your side, lying across the foam roller with your lower leg on the foam roller and heels off the floor.
- The upper leg helps assist balance as you roll the foam roller from the hip joint down to the knee.

Starting position and action

- Lie face down over the foam roller and support your bodyweight on your arms.
- Position the foam roller laterally to your pubic bone on your thigh.
- Slowly roll the foam roller down the outside of your thigh towards your knee.

Shoulder girdle and chest

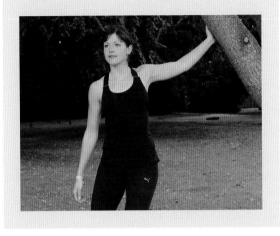

Upper back

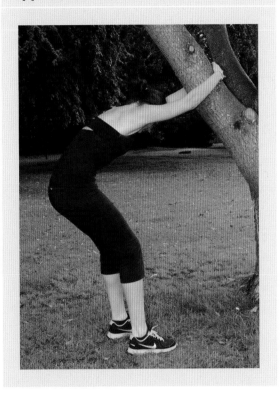

Starting position and action

- Stand next to a doorway, wall or tree and place your left hand or forearm against it, keeping your arm bent but at an angle of approximately 135 degrees.
- Keeping relaxed, slowly turn away from your right arm, to increase the stretch across your chest.
- Hold the stretch position for 10–20 seconds and then repeat, this time with your left arm against the wall and turning to your right side.
- Vary the height of your hand position to vary the stretch you feel through the muscles in the shoulder girdle and chest.
- If you still feel tight, repeat the stretch on both sides.

Starting position and action

- Stand upright and hold on to a post or railing, or if at home, use a secure door handle or similar with both hands level with your chest.
- Holding the post at arms' length, sit back and pull away from the post so that you feel a stretch in your back muscles.
- Hold stretch for 15–20 seconds and repeat.

Triceps

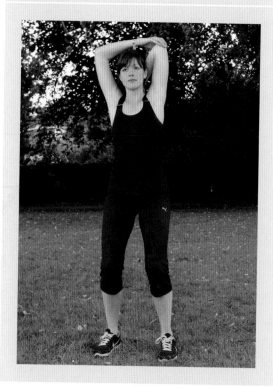

Starting position and action

- Stand upright and lift your right arm upwards with your elbow bent and pointing to the ceiling.
- Use your left hand to assist this stretch by pulling back on your right elbow with your right hand by your right shoulder, holding for 10–15 seconds before repeating, this time stretching your left upper arm.

Hip-flexor stretch

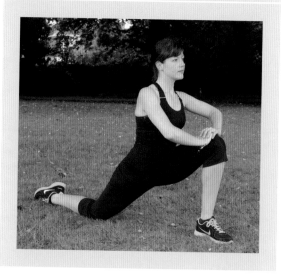

Starting position and action

- From a kneeling position, place your right leg forward so that your thigh is parallel to the floor and your knee is bent at a right angle.
- With your left knee on the floor, lean forward from the hips so that you sink into a hip flexor stretch of the left leg and hold for 15–30 seconds.
- Reach up with your left arm and lean slightly to your right to enhance the stretch.
- Lower your arm and change legs, taking your left leg forward and kneeling on your right knee to repeat the stretch.
- Repeat each stretch 1–3 times.
- As you lean, try and tilt the pelvis under to really focus on stretching the hip flexor muscle.

Hamstrings

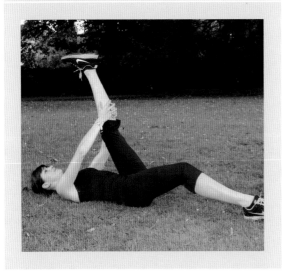

Starting position and action

- Lie on your back with both knees slightly bent and lift your right leg to grasp behind your right thigh.
- Pull gently on your thigh to draw the leg to a stretched position so that you feel tightness on the stretch position.
- Hold this stretched position for 20–30 seconds before releasing and repeating with your left leg.

Quads

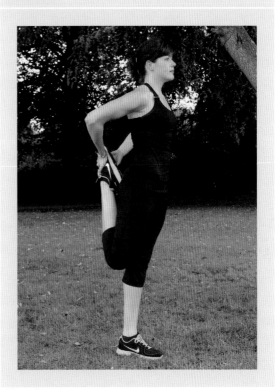

Starting position and action

- Stand up and take hold of your right ankle with your right hand in front of you before extending through your hip to take your right thigh into a stretched position, with your heel behind you against your buttocks.
- Hold this position for 20–30 seconds before repeating with your left leg.

Gastrocnemius

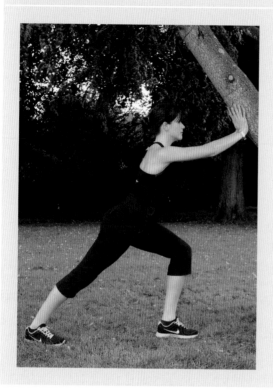

Soleus

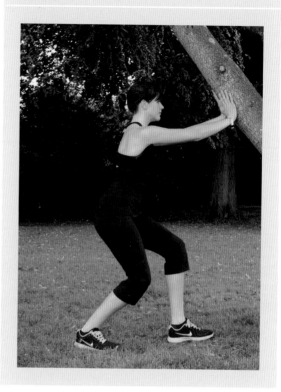

Starting position and action

- From a standing position, push your right leg back behind you with your toes pointing forwards and your heel down to increase the stretch on your calf muscles.
- Hold this stretch position for 15–20 seconds before changing your leg position and repeating.

Starting position and action

- In a standing position similar to the gastrocnemius stretch, with your right leg back and toes pointing forwards, bend your right knee and aim to push it forwards toward the ground, keeping your right heel and foot still to increase the stretch around your ankle. This will stretch both your Achilles tendon and soleus muscle.
- Hold stretch for 15–20 seconds before repeating with your left leg.

GLOSSARY

Absolute strength The maximum amount of force of which a muscle is capable

Aerobic In the presence of oxygen

Agonist The muscle responsible for the movement within an exercise

Anaerobic Without oxygen

Antagonist The opposing muscle to the agonist, within an exercise

ATP This is the chemical energy stored within the muscle cells. It is the breaking down of ATP that releases the energy for muscular activity

Autogenic inhibition A reflex muscular relaxation that occurs in the muscle when the Golgi tendon organ is stimulated (*see also* Golgi tendon organ)

Cardiovascular system The heart, lungs, blood and blood vessels

Cardiac output The total volume of blood pumped by the heart in one minute

Dynamic Balance Controlling your body position while unstable or during movement

Endurance training Performing aerobic exercise at moderate intensities for prolonged periods to create a training effect

Fascia A tough sheet of fibrous tissue supporting and separating skeletal muscles

Foam roller This is a cylindrical foam tube, used to assist Self-Myofascial Release exercises

Functional integration The involvement of all nerves, muscles, joints and ligaments working together to perform a specific movement (*see also* total body integration)

Functional strength The relative strength achieved when applying a force while replicating the body position and movement relative to a specific sporting action

Giant sets A combination of three or more exercises performed as a complete set

Golgi tendon organ A sensory receptor found near the junction of tendons and muscles, which is sensitive to increased tension within the muscle

Holistic therapy Used in the form of fitness training, it involves training muscles and movement as a whole rather than specifically

Integrated functional unit The collective outcome of related muscles, nerves and bones working together in synergy to create a specific movement

Isolation exercise An exercise or movement focussing on a specific muscle or muscle group

Kinetic chain The result of muscles, tendons, ligaments, fascia, nerves and bones working together in synergy

Lumbo-pelvic–hip complex The group of muscles, nerves and bones that are involved in movement and stabilisation around the hips, pelvis and lumbar spine

Mitochondria Often referred to as the 'powerhouse' of a cell, they help produce ATP (*see also* ATP) from organic matter within the cell

Motor skill The ability to co-ordinate movements of joints, muscles and limbs to perform a particular task

Movement pattern The spatial movement relative to the specific exercise or activity

Multi-planar movement Movement involving more than one plane of motion or movement that involves the sagittal, frontal and/or transverse plane

Muscular imbalances When one muscle is overly strong in comparison to a weaker localised muscle

Neuromuscular adaptation When nerves and muscles adapt to the loads, movement and stimuli placed upon them

Neuromuscular efficiency The ability of the neuromuscular system to allow agonists, synergists, stabilisers and neutralisers to work together as an integrated functional unit

Neutraliser The muscle that prevents unwanted movements from another to allow specific alternative movements to occur

Normal length The optimum length of a muscle relative to its normal training movement requirement

Periodisation The process of structuring training into specific periods

Peripheral heart action circuit A workout that generally follows an upper-body exercise with a lower-body exercise, with minimal rest or recovery between the two

Posterior chain The muscles that run down your lower back and legs, including the lower back muscles, glutes, hamstrings and calves

Progressive overload Increasing the resistance as a muscle adapts during a training programme

Proprioception The communication of messages between nerves, muscles and the brain to determine body position, movement and balance

Overspeed training Using elasticated resistance aids or gravity (when running downhill) to assist run speed so neurological adaptation occurs

Reactive balance Exercises that aim to challenge the neuromuscular responses to a change in body position and landing forces, such as recovering from a jump or leap

Stabiliser The muscle that contracts to hold a joint stationary or to minimise movement from another muscle or joint to allow specific alternative movement to occur

Self-myofascial release (SMR) A stretching technique that can improve the flexibility around a joint by applying pressure to stretch receptors within the muscle, which reduces muscle tension and allows increased movement

Stroke volume The volume of blood pumped from the heart with each beat

Super-set Two or more sets of an exercise to work the same or different muscles

Synergistic dominance This occurs when a muscle or group of muscles is weak. Synergists take over the function of the agonists to assist a specific movement (*see also* agonists and synergists)

Synergy Balance between muscles and/or joints

Tendons Bundles of collagen fibres connecting muscles to bones

Total body integration The involvement of all nerves, muscles, joints and ligaments in performing a specific movement (*see also* functional integration)

Variable resistance The resistance varies during the movement, as in the case of resistance tubes, where the resistance increases as the tube is stretched

REFERENCES AND FURTHER READING

REFERENCES

[1] Schurman, C. and Schurman, D., *The Outdoor Athlete* (Human Kinetics, 2009)

[2, 3, 4, 9, 20, 21] Boyle, M., *Advances in Functional Training: Training Techniques for Coaches, Personal Trainers and Athletes* (On Target Publications, 2010)

[5] Musnick, M.D. and Pierce, A.T.C., *Conditioning for Outdoor Fitness, Functional Exercise and Nutrition for Everybody: 2nd Edition* (The Mountaineers Books, 2004)

[6, 7] Bean, A., *The Complete Guide to Strength Training: 3rd Edition* (A& C Black, 2005)

[8] Chek, P., *Movement that Matters* (CHEK Institute, 2000)

[9, 14] Cook, G., *Athletic Body in Balance: Optimal Movement Skills and Conditioning for Performance* (Human Kinetics, 2003)

[10, 11, 13, 19] Clark, M., *Integrated Training for the New Millennium* (National Academy of Sports Medicine, 2000)

[15, 16, 17] Boyle, M., *Functional Training for Sports* (Human Kinetics, 2004)

[18] Foran, B., *High Performance Sports Conditioning* (Human Kinetics, 2001)

[22, 23] Collins, P., *Functional Fitness: Build Your Fittest Body Ever* (Meyer and Meyer Sport, 2009)

[24, 25] Russell, A. and Wallace, T., *Self-Myofascial Release Techniques: Articles – Continuing Education.* (National Academy of Sports Medicine, 2002)

FURTHER READING

Bean, A., *The Complete Guide to Strength Training* (A&C Black, 2005)

Bellomo, D., *Kettlebell Training for Athletes.* (McGraw-Hill, 2010)

Boyle, M., *Advances in Functional Training* (On Target Publications, 2010)

Boyle, M., *Functional Training for Sports* (Human Kinetics, 2004)

Chek, P., *Movement that Matters* (C.H.E.K Institute, 2000)

Chu, D., *Jumping into Plyometrics* (Human Kinetics, 1992)

Collins, P., *Functional Fitness* (Meyer and Meyer Sport, 2009)

Cook, G., *Athletic Body in Action* (Human Kinetics, 2003)

Foran, B., *High Performance Sports Conditioning* (Human Kinetics, 2001)

Hope, B. and Lawrence, M., *The Complete Guide to Circuit Training* (A&C Black, 2002)

Kovacs, M., *Dynamic Stretching* (Ulysses Press, 2010)

Lauren, M., *You Are Your Own Gym* (Ballantine Books, 2011)

Lawrence, M., *The Complete Guide to Core Stability* (A&C Black, 2011)

Murphy, S., *Get Fit Walking* (A&C Black, 2006)

Murphy, S., *The Official British Army Fitness Guide* (Guardian Books, 2009)

Musnick, D. and Pierce, M., *Conditioning for Outdoor Fitness* (The Mountaineers Books, 2004)

Schurman, C and Shurman, D., *The Outdoor Athlete* (Human Kinetics, 2009)

INDEX

suspended bodyweight training
  drills 118, 123, 128, 132, 136–7,
    189–95
  equipment for 42, 44
synergistic dominance 10
synergy 39

T
training
  distance 4
  endurance 40
  functional 8–11
  guidelines 39
  interval 3–4, 39, 53–4
  marathon 54–6
  mid-distance 4
  overspeed 150–3

  resistance 4–6
  sprint 4
trim trails 216–23
tyre drills 154–9

U
urban workouts 141

V
variable resistance 4
ViPR 43
  drills 160–77

W
walking 50–1
warming up 14–27, 52
weight control 41

ACKNOWLEDGEMENTS

In putting this book together, I would firstly like to thank Charlotte and the team at Bloomsbury for their patience and belief that I could attempt such a book and do it justice. In addition I need to thank the production team and trainers who have yet again helped me out in a very demanding photo shoot schedule: Simon, Leighton, Russell, Claire, Sophie and Michelle – many thanks. Grant, once more you have surpassed yourself with the photo shoot – thanks again for being so professional and accommodating with regards to the extent and diversity of photos and venues.

My biggest thank you goes to my family; thank you Michelle for putting up with lost weekends for the past few months and very little family time as a result of the disruption caused by my seemingly endless writing. The two little people I need to thank the most, and also apologise to, are my beautiful, darling children, Sienna and Summer – I promise that should I ever write another book I will absolutely factor in time to play with you, as I know that despite all my writings on outdoor activities and exercise, the irony is that all you wanted to do was play outside in the park. Next time, my little sweethearts, Daddy will make time to play… promise.